# Get Well Soon

Kirsty Mills

The conversations in this book all come from the author's recollections,
though they are not intended to represent word-for-word transcripts.

To Mum, Dad, and Emily.

# FOREWORD

***What this book is not:***

1. A guide for living life with chronic illness.[1] I'm not able to provide groundbreaking wisdom on how I'm living my 'best life' despite my body deciding to go off-piste, because I'm still very much figuring it out as I go along. Rest assured, this book contains no wellness lectures, cortisol-busting diet plans or meditative exercises to combat fatigue.

2. A rant. Sure, I have a few hefty medical conditions that often have a negative impact on my life, and I get pissed off having to deal with them. But I've been lucky enough to have led a life full of amazing experiences, too. What's more, these positive opportunities have often come about *because* of my illnesses.

3. A humblebrag-laden ramble. My aim is not to parade on

[1] A 'chronic' illness is one that is long-lasting or recurring. It does not typically have a cure.

the world stage as if to say: *Look at me! Look how much I've managed to do, despite chronic illness! Am I not just the best thing since wheels on a suitcase?* If anything, over the next 200-ish pages you will learn that I closely resemble a walking buffet of insecurity. I'm contradictory, sometimes jealous, and unsettled, with a side-serving of low self-esteem.[2] My signature scent is that of fading ambition and wasted potential, with top notes of Dolce & Gabbana's 'Light Blue'. So whilst I've managed to succeed in some areas of my life, there's still a lot of work on the personal development side to be done.

4. A misguided attempt to speak on behalf of all patients. There is no one-size-fits-all version of chronic illness; everyone's situation is unique, with different lived experiences from which to contextualise health issues. There may be commonalities, for sure, but illness is highly individualistic. Just as no two bodies are the same, no two experiences of the same illness will align.

Some people might think I've got nothing to complain about. They might assume things can't be that bad if I am able to hold down a job, go dating, do Pilates and fly abroad. Having spent time with people whose health conditions affect them in terrible ways (and thereby having a better understanding of how my own condition could be so much worse) even *I* sometimes think I've not got much to complain about. But there are no Suffering Olympics with gold medals for those living through the most adverse conditions. This account is therefore only a reflection on my experience.

---

[2] I do have *some* redeeming features, though. Promise.

***What this book is:***

At time of writing, I'm a 33-year-old woman who works full time, is followed by a grand total of 189 Instagram users, and has deleted (then re-downloaded) Hinge[3] more times than Rafiki could shake his stick at. I also happen to have a couple of heavy-duty health conditions: liver disease and lupus. Put simply, these are two Ls that nobody has ever put on their wish list for Santa.

Whilst I'll cover these in more detail later, for now I'll say that they're conditions which even Gregory House would baulk at. They both involve my immune system getting a bit confused. Instead of attacking invaders, like it's supposed to, my immune system attacks my own body. Thanks to these diseases, I will likely need a new organ in the not-too-distant future. I will also never see another day on this Earth without downing pills to slow down or counteract the damage these two Ls are inflicting on my body. What's more, some of these medicines make me "immunosuppressed[4]", and come with side-effects that cause other health problems, too.

What I hope to provide is an honest account of the last decade as a millennial with a menagerie of health woes. The book should probably come with a big trigger warning – we'll cover issues such as infertility, hair loss, medical trauma and blood, to name but a few – but I can't *not* include these topics, because they make up the reality of my situation.

I write this book with implicit acknowledgement of my privileges. There are too many to mention, but top picks include a stellar support network (comprising friends, family,

---

[3] For the unacquainted, a dating app.

[4] Immunosuppressant medicines reduce inflammation and weaken your immune system, therefore making you more prone to infections.

and medical professionals), and my luck in being born in a country where healthcare is free at the point of use. These privileges provide a solid foundation from which I can build resilience. I'm all too aware that these privileges are not necessarily afforded to others.

There aren't many books out there about living with chronic illness (I should know, as I've been looking for them), and fewer still *funnier* ones. I write openly for the sake of authenticity, but understand that the humour in my writing might, at times, seem a little jarring given the seriousness of the subject matter. I don't intend to be facetious; this is simply a representation of my attitude to life.

I'm now so used to dealing with serious things that I am able to – and indeed, often need to – approach them through this more light-hearted paradigm. When I'm being told bad health news, or about to be wheeled through for a scary procedure, there's a part of me that is squirreling away all the wee details – the way the doctor stares into the middle distance when thinking, or how badly the paint is peeling from the wall behind the ultrasound machine – and trying to imagine how I'll churn this through the laptop later on. Writing is, and always has been, a powerful tool with which I process my life.

The millennial generation is arguably one of the first to fully benefit from the medical advances of the 21st Century. Many people my age with chronic illness can go about their daily lives thanks to drugs which have only recently been discovered. Had we been born a couple of decades prior, those lives may have been cut short or be of a greatly reduced quality. Yet whilst we are immensely privileged to have these treatments, we also face the challenge of being one of the first generations to balance chronic illness with the expectations and pressures of a fast-paced and uber-competitive world that doesn't place much value on rest. It sometimes feels like there's an overwhelming number of opportunities ripe for the picking, which is only all well and good if you're healthy enough to actually *do* any picking.

If you're not healthy enough, then the ready-made comparison machines in our pockets will happily tell us at any hour of the day that we're not side-hustling/earning /socialising/achieving enough, either. It is quite a time to be alive with chronic illness, and there's not one aspect of my life which isn't impacted in some way by my health.

This book is for anyone – millennial or otherwise – who has woken up in the middle of the night, Googling 'symptoms of sepsis' before proceeding to travel down a wormhole of anxiety. It's for those of us who paint a brave face on, day in and day out, even when we're dreading the results of our latest blood tests. It's for those whose response to being asked '*how are you doing?*' is either '*very well, thanks*' (i.e. I'm not in pain and had a solid eight hours' sleep) or '*not too bad*' (i.e. just finished a fortnight's course of antibiotics, about to start treatment for my ninth thrush infection this year, and waiting for biopsy results to rule out cancer). It's the book I wish had been available to read as a freshly diagnosed teenager, where this new world of hospital appointments was intimidatingly foreign and my future felt increasingly bleak.

Everyone's got 99 problems, it's just that for many people, a health condition ain't one. By its very nature, chronic illness pushes bodies to the limit. More covertly, it pushes souls to their limits, too. In doing so, ill health can bring out aspects of a person that may not otherwise have been realised. Chronic illness has shown me what it means to be human, and it's with that understanding that I trust my reflections can resonate universally. With that in mind, this book is also for anyone who has had a dream that they had to adjust or abandon; for anyone who has felt powerless or resentful at the way their life has played out; and for anyone who has struggled to keep positive in a seemingly hopeless situation.

Unfortunately, there is no real-life Glinda the Good waiting to float down in a bubble of anti-bac, promising to wave a wand and magic away problems, health-related or otherwise. That said, I hope that my account can be a bit like a word hug that lets you know that you're not the only one going through challenging times. You're never alone. Or at least, you're not alone in feeling alone. Maybe these words might give you the confidence to reflect upon, and feel a little more comfortable in, your own ability to face difficult situations. If nothing else, I hope it gives you a laugh. After all, laughter is the best medicine.[5]

(P.S. Whilst I've tried to be thorough in my research and editing, I apologise for any errors in medical terminology or explanations. Corrections are openly encouraged.)

(P.P.S. Nothing in this book should be considered medical advice. Always seek professional help. And by 'professional help', I mean a GP, not a Paltrow-esque shaman on Instagram.)

---

[5] We're already cracking open the clichés!

# ON THE SOUNDTRACK OF A LIFE WITH CHRONIC ILLNESS

Nibbling through the last two chunks of a half-melted bar of chocolate in my car, I flipped through the NHS-endorsed '*Managing Stress*' booklet that had been distributed at work earlier that day. Its top coping mechanisms to combat 'feelings of overwhelm' were:

- Eating well
- Sleeping well
- Getting out in nature
- Meditation and/or alternative nostril breathing
- Taking a break and having a KitKat[6]

I stuffed the booklet into my glove compartment along with the chocolate wrapper. Disappointingly, but not altogether

[6] OK, this last one was not in the booklet. I made it up.

surprisingly, the book didn't contain coping mechanisms for when you've been told, at 31 years of age, that you potentially have a hip condition requiring a full-blown joint replacement.

Ten minutes earlier, I was lying back on a sports therapy clinic bed, with the distance between my flopped-out knees and the horizontal being measured by a physiotherapist.

"So, it's 23 centimetres on that side, which is totally normal." He motioned to my right hip. "And on the left, we have…" He paused, twisting his head to read the tape more easily, "…well, we have, eh, *12 centimetres.*"

I screwed my face up at the Artex ceiling. "Quite a difference, then."

"Have a seat," he said, dashing towards the PC to input the measurements before he forgot the numbers, his fingers pausing from their rapid-fire dance across the keyboard only to push acetate-framed glasses an inch or so further up the bridge of his nose. Wincing discreetly, I contorted my body off the bed and plunged into the chair.

Seven weeks of the Couch-to-5k fitness programme over winter had left me hobbling with hip pain. When I was still struggling to walk despite a fortnight's rest, I scheduled a physiotherapist appointment and rued the day I thought getting fit was a good idea.

"So, the thing is, if you were any other person your age with the same symptoms, I would tell you to go away, do these exercises, and come back to see me in a month if it's still sore," he said.

"Right."

"But…" he began. *Hark!* The sweet sound of a 'but': the conjunction of doom, the harbinger of shattered illusions. "…you're not like any other 30-something."

He flashed the briefest of smiles, as though this was something resembling a compliment. He wasn't wrong, *per se.* I'm not like most other 30-somethings. It's not that I possess ethereal, traffic-halting levels of beauty. I don't have a secret million-pound crypto fund listed on the FTSE. Nobel Peace Prize-winning crusader for human rights, I am not. Alas, what sets me apart is my medical history, or as I like to call it, *War and Peace 2: The Sequel Nobody Asked For.* It's my tangled web of disorders and diseases which extends some way beyond any tale of Russian destitution that Tolstoy could dream up.

The smile morphed into a frown as he began speaking again. "It could be that your hip pain is caused by something called *avascular necrosis.*"

My brain sparked off a desperate hunt for clues. This potential diagnosis wasn't something I'd anticipated hearing. I'd been caught off-guard.

*Avascular* didn't sound very pretty. Probably something to do with blood or veins. Circulation, maybe.

*Necrosis* sounded positively awful. Based on my limited knowledge of medical etymology, I was 99% certain that this meant 'death'. Necromancer, necropolis, necrophil – nah, nothing good ever comes from a word beginning with 'necro'.

There's a phrase which I tend to use in times like these, and that phrase is 'fuckity-fuck'. If I'm on my own, I'll say it aloud with emphasis on the 'f' for extra catharsis. If I'm in polite company, I'll make do with it playing out on the ticker tape in my mind. This was shaping up to be a top-tier (silent) fuckity-fuck moment.

"Oh. Doesn't sound very good," I said with a delivery that could have been in the running for understatement of the year.

"Basically, it's a condition where the blood supply is cut off to the hip bone. And then the hip bone dies." We both sat in silence for a beat. "Now, it's important to keep in mind that it might not be this, because it's very rare, so it's probably, possibly, maybe, *not* avascular necrosis. But I'd prefer to get it ruled out to be on the safe side, because avascular necrosis can happen if you've been taking steroids[7] for a long time, which you have been. And it's more common in people who have lupus, like you. Again, it might be absolutely nothing, but –"

"But I have a tendency to attract rare things." I finished his sentence, trying to wrangle my Doc Martens back on without inducing a stabbing pain. Maybe I should have been more accurate in my statement: I accumulate *bad* rare things, mostly in the way of medical diagnoses, rather than *good* rare things like lottery wins, artefacts that are impressive enough to be shown to Fiona Bruce in the Antiques Roadshow, or meet-cutes in Parisian cafés with tall, dark, handsome men. "And what's the treatment, if it is this avascular…thingy?"

He grimaced. "Surgery. A hip replacement."

*Fuckity-fuck-fuck-fuck.*

A week after the physiotherapist appointment, I had an X-

[7] Corticosteroids are a type of immunosuppressant. Note that my steroids are not the same ones which give you muscles like Arnold Schwarzenegger.

ray which ruled out the advanced stages of avascular necrosis (this was good news). But the X-ray also detected a less-serious condition called hip impingement, which might make me prone to arthritis (slightly bad news).

A week after *that*, I had a routine ultrasound scan of my abdomen – more on why I get those later – which showed I had not only an 'angry-looking' gallbladder (not great news) but also increased amounts of fluid around my liver (far from ideal news, and quite unexpected), with a spleen the size of a juicy mango when it should be an avocado (not wonderful news in the slightest, but expected).

My doctor emailed me a week later to inform me that, on closer inspection of the ultrasound scan, there were signs of small veins in my stomach lining leaking blood. This is caused by having a poorly liver. The doctor advised my annual endoscopy[8] be brought forward to check things out.

During this same timeframe, I:

1. Started a new job in a completely new industry with zero knowledge of anything.
2. Broke up with yet another Hinge match who I hoped would be a bit more long-term, but ended up being thrown overboard from the situationship.
3. Was diagnosed with the holy trifecta of genitourinary infections (a UTI[9], bacterial vaginosis[10], *and* thrush[11])

---

[8] This procedure is basically when a long, flexible tube (scope) is put down your throat to let doctors see what lurks within. If there are swollen bits of vein (called varices) that look like they're going to bleed, a separate attachment is added onto the scope, and a fancy procedure is done to make the varices less likely to bleed. This is called variceal banding, and I'll talk more about it later. Bet you can't wait.

[9] Urinary tract infection, where bacteria in the urethra (where you pee from) get out of hand and it starts to feel like you're pissing razor blades.

[10] A bacterial imbalance of the vagina, the cause of which is unclear, because y'know, women's health is still a bit of a mystery.

[11] Overgrowth of yeast in the vagina. Yay.

which made my pee smell like the waste stream from a sulphur generation plant. I was prescribed antibiotics and Canesten. Unfortunately, being immunosuppressed means infections like these can be really common.

4. Deleted Hinge, reinstalled Hinge, swiped my way through the 35 men without an evident red flag in my 55-mile radius, decided Hinge's Nobel Prize-winning algorithm was seriously flawed, and then reinstalled Bumble (another equally depressing dating app).
5. Researched local convents, only to find the nearest one would involve relocation to England. Deciding I liked Scottish tap water too much, I scratched the idea.

The advice in the stress booklet is useful, I suppose, if you have the anxiety level of a goldfish. It's somewhat less helpful when your baseline anxiety hovers around the 'hope-my-organ-doesn't-fail-today' mark. The reality is that the events I've described above aren't particularly out of the ordinary for me, because chronic illness is a lifelong soundtrack. It's something mildly sombre (I'm thinking early 00s' David Gray) and once it starts playing, it can't ever be muted. Some days it's a little quieter than others, but there's always a din underpinning every decision, every moment of happiness, every disappointment, and every life milestone.

There will be times that the background hum is welcomed, because it provides a certain harmony, or a bit of perspective, to the clashing noise going on in other parts of your life (because, of course, none of the other life stuff magically disappears just because you've got health woes to be preoccupied with). Other times it becomes so obtrusively, overwhelmingly loud that, no matter how much I wish I could escape the cacophony, I can't. Whilst I will never get used to it being there, humming away, I equally can't remember my life without it.

There are times when it is possible to forget about my health and live resolutely 'in the moment'. I'll actively decide not to think about the new bruises that appeared on my forearm overnight, or won't look in the mirror when I don my wig in the morning. I'll go for a walk along the beach and not retreat into a negative thought spiral when I pass the playpark and remember that I'm not able to have biological children.

There are echoes of the bright-eyed, teenaged ingénue in the motivated, sensitive and generally optimistic 30-something version of me. Deep down, I'm still the girl I was before I emerged into the world of repeat prescriptions and butterfly needles, hospital department bingo and scopes in orifices I never imagined anyone would need to see. And it's from that safe haven of naivety that we're going to kick off the story in earnest.

# ON THE ROAD TO DIAGNOSIS (EVERYTHING'S GOING PETE TONG BUT NOBODY KNOWS WHY, SO YOU'RE PINBALLED TO TEN SPECIALISTS)

Being a proud geek, I love a statistic. Here's one that's equally shocking and, to those of us living on the autoimmune rollercoaster, completely unsurprising: on average, it takes *five years* for a person to receive a diagnosis of autoimmune disease. During this time, patients will see an average of six doctors.[i] Now, because there is nothing more boring than someone droning on about a medical diagnosis 'journey', I'll try to keep mine fairly snappy. But even the potted summary is bamboozling.

With no doubt about it, my childhood was full of *Little House on the Prairie*-level wholesomeness. My sister and I were cocooned with home-cooked meals, after-school Brownies and weekends spent perfecting Steps' dance routines. The family tree, fastidiously researched to eight generations by my father, was generally healthy: no history of cancer, diabetes, liver problems, or obvious autoimmune conditions. Between them, my grandparents were prescribed three medications; my mother would only consider downing a paracetamol if her leg happened to be impaled on a fence. We were all fit specimens, thank you very much.

Healthy, that is, except for my lack of regular periods.[12] By my mid-teens, I had only had a handful of long, heavy bleeds, with months between them. Unusual, perhaps, but Mum had started her periods around sixteen, and my Granny later still. I thought my cycle was just having commitment issues, but was nonetheless dragged by my parents to see a GP.

This GP initially suspected anorexia, until Mum politely confirmed I was partial to a fish supper every Friday night. I proceeded to show the doctor a couple of blotchy red veins that had appeared on my upper arms. Spider veins[13], as I now know them to be, are dilated blood vessels with smaller leakages around the circumference of a central spot, giving the appearance of a spider's web on the skin. The GP took a quick look and described them – so clearly in my memory, almost two decades later – as a 'cosmetic' problem. If they really bothered me, I could have them injected with a vein-clearing agent…but that would not be available on the NHS.

Somewhat satisfied with the GP's conclusion that my periods would even out when exam stress was over, we left the clinic and happily bought into the concept that we were worrying over nothing. I now know that both amenorrhea and spider veins can be symptoms of advanced liver disease.

---

[12] To use the fancy medical term, *amenorrhea*.

[13] Also known as *telangiectasias*. You can see why they're nicknamed 'spider veins'.

The point of this tale is not to summon a witch hunt against the GP (those who indulge in GP-bashing are often the same people who failed Standard Grade Biology). I do not retrospectively accuse the doctor, with my benefit of hindsight, of being insufficiently thorough in their investigations. My symptoms were so insidious, and my liver condition so rare, that the doctor was quite within their right to assume that the problems were unconnected and the cause innocuous.

By the same token, perhaps Mum and I should have been more persistent, and demanded more tests. Today, after hundreds of appointments with doctors and being significantly more medically versed, I feel better placed to self-advocate. My mother blames herself for not pushing more, for not taking me back to the doctor against my will, and I only wish I could absolve her of that misplaced guilt.[14]

Spending energy and time today ruminating on the GP's judgement is futile; we are where we are. A constructive takeaway would perhaps be to ensure that doctors – and moreover, the public – are aware of the subtler signs of liver damage.

I pushed the dodgy periods to the back of my mind until reaching university in Edinburgh. I don't know why it took me so long to follow up on this – probably a combination of not wanting anything to distract me from studies and not wanting

---

[14] Mum also questions whether she did, or didn't do, something when we were growing up that would have led to my conditions. Was she right to let me get the HPV jab? Should she have not let me eat chocolate? Should she have intervened when I was getting stressed over exams? As much as I tell her that, if anything, her resolute commitment to providing us with a secure childhood has given me the skills with which to lead a healthy life and manage my conditions, I know there is a part of her that will never not blame herself and it makes me very sad.

to make a fuss – and whilst I try not to blame myself, it is one of my few regrets. In my second term at university, I noticed I was losing more hair than normal in the shower, and this scared me enough to go to the GP in Edinburgh.

I recall sitting down on a rickety plastic chair whilst balancing a clipboard on my crossed knee to diligently complete the university GP practice's new patient form. *Any medical history?* Suspected asthma as a child, which had resolved. *Current medication?* N/A. I had taken no drugs other than a couple batches of antibiotics. *Allergies?* Feeling a bit boring having no medical history of interest, I wrote what I always wrote on these types of forms under the allergies section: blue food colouring. Why I thought this was relevant, I'm not quite sure; perhaps if there was an inexplicable medical intervention requiring an intravenous drip of M&Ms, I'd be doomed. On reflection, these were the halcyon days. Except that they never really were, because I was unknowingly hosting a diseased liver and a wayward immune system.

The GP at the Edinburgh practice, a taciturn Irishman in an elbow-padded tweed jacket and a chaotic desk to match, scribbled some hieroglyphics with a bleeding fountain pen as I relayed off my symptoms. I was sent away for blood tests.

The blood tests showed that I had a slightly raised level of a specific hormone, which, when combined with the lack of periods and hair loss, led to a diagnosis of **polycystic ovary syndrome.**[15] There wasn't much follow-up on this; I was handed a couple of leaflets and told that help would be available if I wanted to conceive in future.

---

[15] Abbreviated to PCOS.

The blood tests also flagged low levels of platelets[16] and I was therefore added to a haematology[17] waiting list. Months later, a haematologist diagnosed me with my first autoimmune condition, **immune thrombocytopenia**[18] (try saying *that* before your morning coffee). Simplistically, this means that the immune system starts destroying the body's own platelets. The consultant said it wouldn't be a problem unless I was in a car crash or giving birth. As neither of these was on my immediate to-do list, and the platelet levels weren't insanely low, there was no further action required other than routine blood tests to keep an eye on things.

Then a few months later, *another* routine blood test flagged up *another* dodgy result which led to *another* referral, this time to rheumatology[19], who then told me I had *another* autoimmune condition called **lupus.**[20]

The term 'autoimmune' is being bandied around here like it's common parlance, when to some lucky ducks out there, it's not. To explain very simplistically (and I'm not a medic so take this description, researched as it is, with a pinch of salt): the body has an innate 'immune system'. This system comprises a complex set of biological processes which are designed to work together like a little defence army within the body. The army's job is to ensure that any virus or pathogen (basically anything which is foreign to the body and has the potential to cause harm) is destroyed or, at the very least, conquered down to a level which makes it safe to live with. Whilst some smart scientists *kinda* understand how the immune system works, nobody fully comprehends all its intricacies.

---

[16] Platelets are a component of your blood that helps it to clot.

[17] Branch of medicine involving blood conditions.

[18] Abbreviated to ITP.

[19] Specialist for conditions causing pain or inflammation in the joints, muscles, bones and tissues.

[20] Otherwise known as systemic lupus erythematosus, abbreviated to SLE.

The added complication lies in that every person's immune system is slightly different, just like their DNA, or Netflix recommendations. We know, for example, that sometimes the immune system army goes rogue, SAS-style, and doesn't follow the standard operating procedure. A good example of this is allergies. When someone is allergic to, say, peanuts, then what is happening (again, simplistically) is that the body's immune system misidentifies the peanut as public enemy number one and so mounts an overly dramatic response to the slightest whiff of a Snickers bar. The defence tactics – potentially a lethal anaphylactic shock – are nowhere near proportionate to the danger the Snickers bar presented in the first place.

Autoimmune disease, then, is essentially where the body's immune system army messes up big time and starts something of a civil war. The immune system starts to attack the body it's meant to be defending, rather than the invaders. There are many autoimmune conditions that you've maybe already heard of, including rheumatoid arthritis, Crohn's disease, and type 1 diabetes. Unfortunately, most autoimmune conditions – their causes, the factors influencing disease progression, and the treatment options – are poorly understood.

Autoimmune patients usually experience 'flares' of their illness, where symptoms get worse, in between periods of 'remission', where the disease is still present, but symptoms are lessened. My flares tend to be triggered by having a cold or another infection which then ramps up my immune response. My immune system then gets a bit too high on its own supply and kicks off a flare.

Lupus patients can present with myriad problems including aches, pains, fatigue, rashes, neurological symptoms, gastrointestinal irregularities, organ failure, and spontaneous third ear growth.[21] Essentially, the body starts attacking its own healthy tissues. The classic signs are joint pain and a butterfly-shaped rash over the cheeks. Ready for a fun fact? The term 'lupus' is attributed to a 13th Century physician called Rogerius. Rogerius used it to describe lupus' erosive facial lesions on patients, which he felt were reminiscent of wolf bites. The Latin word for wolf is lupus.[ii] Rogerius' way with words was no doubt reflective of a delightful bedside manner.

Now, my body doesn't like doing anything by the book, so these typical lupus symptoms were never really part of my repertoire. Instead, I was diagnosed with the combination of hair loss along with a detectable amount of lupus antibodies in my blood. Together, this was deemed sufficient to confirm with a wobbly degree of certainty that I had a 'lupus-esque' illness (autoimmune conditions are terribly *vague*. The goalposts of diagnosis are often wishy-washy, overlapping, and not well understood). Indeed, even in this book, you'll notice most of my reflections centre around liver disease rather than lupus. This is because I feel that the liver problems have the most direct impact on my life.

To recap (and I forgive you if you're confused at this point, because I was, too; finding out what was wrong with me was more complex than uncovering the Higgs-Boson particle): I was fast becoming a vessel for acronyms, with lupus (SLE), ovary problems (PCOS) and a blood clotting problem (ITP). Bizarre as it might seem, I wasn't too fazed by the slow avalanche of diagnoses, most likely because none of the doctors I met seemed to be *that* concerned. Nothing was immediately life-threatening, and there were treatment options available. Indeed, it felt like these conditions partially explained

[21] I made that last one up, but you get the gist.

the cause of the two symptoms that were worrying me the most: hair loss and lack of periods. Having fancy diagnoses took the edge off the maelstrom of uncertainty.

Being the overachiever I was, I attended all my hospital appointments, somehow fitting them in amongst an increasingly busy life at university. I had more blood drained from me than a character in Twilight, my legs were contorted into questionable positions to test joint mobility, and my bone density was confirmed as excellent, thanks to a misspent youth of trampoline addiction. Ultimately, I was released back into the wild with a follow-up rheumatology appointment and a lifelong prescription for a drug (hydroxychloroquine, the same drug Trump incorrectly advised everyone should take to ward off Covid-19) to slow any future progression of lupus. This, I was told, might also help with my hair loss.

"We tend to find that, if lupus is going to attack any of the organs, it will do so most viciously in the first few years after diagnosis," the rheumatologist declared at our initial consultation. "It doesn't appear to have done much damage to you, so you can take comfort from that." I smiled and nodded, taking the same level of comfort as I would from cosying up next to a porcupine freshly bathed in uranium waste.

Despite hoovering up hydroxychloroquine in the hope that it would stop my hair falling out, months later I was still battling to hide an ever-growing thinning patch on the crown of my head. And then fell the first domino in a chain of events that changed the ball game: a routine blood test just before Christmas 2012 showed a spiked level of a specific liver enzyme.[22]

[22] Alanine Transaminase, or ALT, which is an indicator of liver inflammation.

One afternoon just before New Year, I received a decidedly un-festive phone call from my Edinburgh GP.[23] Because the liver enzyme was so high, I was told to immediately stop taking hydroxychloroquine, my lupus medication, in case it was having a toxic effect on my liver.

The GP had arranged for me to have an ultrasound scan of my liver on my return to Edinburgh, to "check over a few things". Despite thinking I had become a dab hand at joining waiting lists, dampening worries, being ferried between departments and adapting to new medical terminology, I was not prepared in the slightest for what was coming my way. Those 'few things' that needed checked over turned out to be a major turning point in my life.

---

[23] I've since learned that it's usually not a good thing to be called directly by GPs. It probably means you're in dangerous territory.

# ON DIAGNOSIS, PROPER

Weeks later, in the depths of a particularly gloomy February 2013, I was lying flat out in a darkened ultrasound clinic room. A sonologist[24] swept the scanner's probe across my abdomen, rolling it in between the crevices of each of my ribs, pushing a little harder here and a little deeper there to get a clearer picture. It had never before occurred to me quite how many ribs there are in the human body, but I was acutely aware of every single one as the specialist played them like a calcified xylophone. I struggled to contain small reflexive outbursts of laughter – I'm very ticklish – but the silence in the room made it inappropriate to even breathe audibly. The sonologist reaffixed the scanner probe back into its little holder next to the screen.

"When's your next GP appointment?" they asked, pinging their blue gloves off and rolling them into a tight rubber missile for the waste bin.

---

[24] Medical professional who performs ultrasound scans.

"I don't think I've got one," I said. Truth be told, I wasn't entirely sure what the point of the ultrasound was. Nobody had told me I needed to make a GP appointment for afterwards, too.

"Well, you need to phone the clinic today. Tell them you need an appointment tomorrow."

"Is everything ok, or…" My voice trailed off, caught in its own dryness. I hadn't had anything to eat or drink all day, and it was now well past 4pm; my blood sugar levels were plunging.

"I can't discuss the scan. You need to speak to your GP."

I nodded silently, afraid to push further. They opened the door and signalled for me to leave. No 'don't worry', no smile, no 'have a good day'. Nothing.

This new medical world often wasn't very friendly, it certainly wasn't pretty and (judging by the waiting rooms' coffee tables piled high with SAGA magazines) it wasn't brim-full with young people, either. Whilst I was now averaging one medical appointment per fortnight, all I wanted to do was buckle down and concentrate on my third year at university. Thing is, bodies don't work around schedules. And so, in between spending every waking moment in the library prepping for my organic chemistry exams, I made a next-day appointment with the GP.

The GP explained that the ultrasound showed my liver had a degree of damage. I was being referred to gastroenterology[25]

[25] The department for conditions affecting the gastrointestinal tract and associated organs, including the liver. Specialists in liver disease are called hepatologists. 'Hepatic' means 'relating to the liver'.

and also fast-tracked for a liver biopsy.[26]

Despite the Byzantine bureaucracy of the NHS, when there's something *really* wrong, stuff does tend to happen quickly. In fact, the urgency of the ultrasound and then the liver biopsy – all within a matter of weeks – was a bit bewildering in comparison to the months-long waits for previous referrals. The difference in tone was marked; I sensed something was amiss.

Sure enough, within a fortnight of the liver biopsy, I sat on a navy-blue plastic chair in a consultant's office at the Royal Infirmary in Edinburgh, chaperoned on either side by my parents, and was told that I had irreversible damage to my liver tissue.

"How much do you drink?" the consultant asked, his pen hovering above a freshly printed questionnaire[27] for new patients.

"Maybe three vodka and limes on a night out. And that's maybe once, twice a month?" I frowned, already feeling that this was too much but knowing that my monthly total was the ski society's definition of an evening's entrée. "It was maybe a couple of times a week when I was in first year of uni. And maybe some shots."

Could drinking be the cause of the damage? The total

---

[26] Biopsies are samples of tissue taken for analysis. A liver biopsy usually involves sucking out a sliver of liver through the side of your body using a long, medieval-looking needle. This is somewhat preferable to the alternative, which is done when the blood clotting factors are not great: threading a biopsy needle through the jugular vein down to get a sample from the liver. The tissue sample is then scrutinised to help identify the specific type of tissue damage.

[27] The NHS loves a questionnaire or nine.

sounded worse when I said it out loud, but it wasn't *that* much, surely? I could count the number of times I had been woozily drunk on two hands, and I had never forgotten parts of a night out due to drink. I hadn't touched alcohol at all in school, choosing instead to be that obtuse *'I'm not like other girls'* girl whose beverage of choice was mineral water at the sixth form afterparty. In what will forever be one of the universe's best jokes, I recall actually thinking that my liver would make a great transplant for someone one day.

"Okay." The doctor cleared his throat. "And I'm aware that your parents are here, and you might not want to discuss this, but…" He threw an apologetic look to my Mum and Dad, as though the next question would risk breaking Omertà, "…have you ever taken illegal drugs?"

I looked him dead in the eye. This man clearly didn't know me, the golden child who had never so much as touched a cigarette. None of my pals dabbled in drugs and as such it had never really been on my radar. Studying chemistry, I was aware of the need for quality control in drug synthesis. The mere thought of ingesting anything that had been reconstituted on a garage floor in South Lanarkshire, only to then be topped up with diluted methylated spirit and finished with a thickening agent of concrete, gave me the beginnings of an anxiety attack.

"No."

"Righto. Just needed to confirm." He ticked off another box on the questionnaire. "It appears, then, that your biopsy results are indicative of a condition called autoimmune hepatitis[28], where your immune system attacks your liver cells, causing inflammation. Based on your liver numbers right now,

[28] Abbreviated to AIH.

you're going through an acute flare of the illness. We'll need to start you on high-dose steroids to suppress that immune response and make your liver better." That word again. Autoimmune. "And regrettably it seems that this condition has already harmed your liver to the extent of what we call cirrhosis."

I struggled to get words out, my mind already struggling to process all this information. "But…the liver can regenerate, right?"

He grimaced. "Not at cirrhosis stage, unfortunately. The inflammation has changed the fundamental architecture of the organ. The tissue is now too scarred to repair itself. You'll have cirrhosis forever, unless you have a liver transplant."

The trouble with being a good student is that my life motto was, and continues to be, *'fail to prepare, prepare to fail'.* Going into that appointment, I'd already done due diligence on liver conditions; I knew that there was a high likelihood I would have autoimmune hepatitis. I just hadn't factored in the cirrhosis bit. It felt disturbing to learn that something so life-threatening had been going on inside my body for an unknown length of time, stealthily eking away at my longevity. I was unwittingly killing myself.

The doctor explained that I'd likely be on medication to suppress my immune system for life, though it was possible for some AIHers to have months or even years without needing much immunosuppression. I could continue being relatively healthy, with my liver functioning well despite the damage, if we were able to prevent my immune system causing further inflammation. Whilst I might need a liver transplant if my liver started to fail, it could be years or maybe even decades down the line. Even then, the AIH might return in the transplanted organ.

"I'm glad we caught this when we did," the doctor added quietly whilst printing off and scribbling over a prescription form. "Often patients with AIH are wheeled into A&E at death's door, requiring an urgent liver transplant. Many don't survive. You are at a more treatable stage."

I nodded. I didn't cry, or ask more questions, or throw myself onto the wipe-clean linoleum floor and kick my feet in a tantrum. I didn't do anything, really, other than to shake his hand again, and say *thank you,* and slip the prescription note in amongst the lecture notes in my satchel, and walk with my parents in humbled silence to pick up a small suitcase of medication from the hospital pharmacy.

The problem with autoimmune conditions is that because nobody can really pinpoint what the trigger is – it could be stress, it could be medication, it could be an environmental external agent along with a genetic predisposition – it makes it so much harder to predict how they'll behave.

Being diagnosed with a chronic illness, especially when you're young, can feel like being marooned on an island from which all escape routes have been sabotaged. Nobody in my support network at the time – none of my friends and none of my family – had anything like the same number of medical issues I now faced. Nobody could relate to how isolating it felt. Whilst the road to diagnosis was protracted and confusing, in many ways I was more adrift at the end than I had felt at the start.

What's more, I soon realised that the diagnosis itself was just the initial wave. Over the following weeks, months and years, the medications, side effects and psychological turmoil crashed the party like unwelcome guests commandeering the Spotify playlist of my life.

# ON HAIR LOSS...

*"Hair,"* in the words of Fleabag, *"is everything"*. She wasn't wrong. Good stylistic arrangement of the dead protein strands sprouting from your head can, through mysterious magic, be the deciding factor between your day having more endorphins than a dancer in the *La La Land* opening sequence, and 24 protracted hours wherein you want to retreat into a dimly lit cave devoid of reflective surfaces. If it was possible to bottle up the confidence emanating from the pores of a woman sporting a blow-dry fresh out the hairdresser, then you can bet your bottom dollar Jeff Bezos would be selling it on Black Friday.

As a youngster, I was 'blessed' with a full-on triangle of frizz which would sometimes, weather-permitting and if Mercury was in retrograde, untangle into something resembling curls. Think of Hagrid in the Harry Potter films, and you wouldn't be far off. I distinctly remember a visit to the hairdresser in my second year of high school. Surveying the frizz situation and deciding that it wasn't worth the effort to calm the curls, she wielded a new weapon (GHDs) to iron out any waves, with the added benefit of making my hair easier to chop. Within a mere 20 minutes, my self-esteem skyrocketed as I watched my transformation into a cool and straightened teenager. Finally, I had the hair I had spent many nights praying to the Gods for.

To keep this charade of sleekness for as long as possible, I didn't wash my hair for three whole days. When I ended up having no option than to shampoo, I did so only on the proviso that I could then use my Mum's straighteners to ward off the merest hint of a wave. Which I proceeded to do, religiously, every single day for the next year. The lack of heat protection spray combined with non-ceramic ironing plates resulted in my hair slowly morphing back, albeit straighter, into a pyramid of frizz.

Presumably cringing at her daughter's straw barnet, my Mum came home one day armed with a bottle of curling mousse from Boots. When massaged into damp hair, this heaven-sent foam transformed my unruly mane into perfectly bouncy, if a little crunchy, ringlets. That's not to say I fully embraced my curls *au naturelle*. I recall tentatively wandering into a chic hairdressing salon in Singapore[29], with July 2007's edition of *Seventeen* magazine lodged firmly under my arm.

"Can I maybe get my hair like that, please?" I asked the hairdresser, flopping the magazine open to the page where I'd turned down the corner to mark a picture of Emma Watson at the third Harry Potter film premiere, sporting glossy, beach-wavy boho curls.

The head stylist looked at Emma, then at me, and then back at the magazine once again. Brandishing his scissors in the air,

---

[29] My dad worked there for a few years when I was a teenager, and we stayed during the school holidays.

their metal blades glistening in the studio's fancy spotlights, he puffed out his cheeks.

"We can try, *lah.*"

What I neglected to tell him, of course, that what I was *really* looking for was for him to transform the other bits of me – the awful acne, translucent skin, prominent nose and worsening overbite – into Emma, too. Alas, he was a hairdresser rather than fully-fledged miracle worker, and it soon transpired that he wasn't particularly skilled at cutting curly hair, either. I decided it was for the best to avoid my reflection whilst he snipped and diffused away.

"What do you think?" he asked, standing back in admiration of his *fait accompli.*

Gazing into the mirror, my eyes cast over the poodle-esque ringlets which seemed to have grown exponentially more bountiful atop my head thanks to a guava-fragranced serum. Having perfected a faux reaction of "*Oh, now this is exactly what I was after, thank you so much*" from years of disappointing hairdressing experiences, I pulled out all the stops for an Oscar-worthy performance. My lips contorted themselves into a rictus grin so wide that it would be better suited to walking up an aisle than the output of a haircut.

After paying my (correction, *my dad's*) S$150 through gritted teeth, I fled the aircon-ed mall into the humidified jungle of Singapore, whereupon my curls puffed out into a seismic frizz bomb as a resounding middle finger to the serum in which they were embalmed. In typical melodramatic teenaged fashion, I flicked away the tears trailing their way down my puppy-fat-rounded cheeks, ignoring concerned looks of passers-by. It was obvious: I could never, ever look as pretty as Emma, and I was stupid to even think that a hairdresser might make my hair look like hers. It's more than a little bittersweet that, 10 years later, I would finally get Emma Watson-level hair…but only after I'd lost most of my own.

When my hair started to fall out during my first term at university, I assigned it to the stress of leaving home and not eating very much to keep my student budget as low as possible (you know you've got a bit of problem when one plain Ryvita and a Penguin biscuit constitutes lunch). I adapted by wearing my hair up in a bun, to avoid the bald spot being visible at the crown. Soon enough, my scalp peeked through the top. More and more hairs swirled round the plughole in the communal shower in halls, which couldn't only be attributed to using the cheapest shampoo from Home Bargains.

As mentioned already, I finally plucked up the courage to visit the Irish GP at the university clinic. Besides referring me for blood tests, he also sent me to a dermatologist[30] to check my hair loss. That dermatology appointment remains, to this day, one of my most distressing clinical experiences.

Not wanting my parents to make the four-hour journey down from the Highlands to join me, I sat alone in the waiting room, mentally analysing every angle of my hopeful expectations that this appointment would be the key that unlocked the mystery of my thinning hair. At that point, I had been told that while PCOS (the ovary condition) was *likely* to be the cause of my hair loss, it was very much a working hypothesis (and I didn't yet know about lupus, either). This 20-minute dermatology slot then, I decided, was going to be an extinguishing foam over the fireball of anxiety that smouldered every single day at the pit of my stomach.

---

[30] Doctor specialising in hair, skin and nails.

Instead, I learned that afternoon that very rarely does a single appointment set the scene for a prettily wrapped-up conclusion. After waiting for over an hour, I was only too happy to be greeted by a slightly eccentric, bowtie-wearing doctor in his late 50s.

"So, you've been sent to me today to take a look at your hair loss, is that right?" He peered up from a folder of papers, sunlight beaming in behind him through frosted-glass windows. I shifted awkwardly in the plastic seat, wondering if I had ever seen anyone wear a bowtie in the flesh before.

"Yes. It's been thinning for maybe over a year now."

"You've already been diagnosed with PCOS, too?"

I nodded.

"I see." Clicking his tongue at the top of his mouth, he narrowed his eyes to scan across my head. "Well, I'll need to take a closer look at the shape of the hair follicles through a microscope."

He cut off a small strip of Sellotape, placing it on my head as a makeshift tool with which to artfully rip a few hairs out. "On the count of three: one, two –" he yanked, I winced, and then a wave of queasiness washed over me at the very real prospect that we (or more specifically, *he)* had just made a bad situation so much worse. As he wandered off to put the sample under the lens, I dug out my pocket mirror to surreptitiously confirm that I didn't now have a Sellotape-wide bald spot on the exact area where I was actively trying to keep as many hairs in place as possible.

"Interesting," he murmured, one eye focussed on the specimen. "Do you mind if I bring a colleague in for a look?"

Wandering over to the door, he returned with another equally old and bespectacled man. They both looked at my scalp, prizing apart the hair on my head, humming and hawing and having a hushed discussion between them.

"Very interesting indeed," the second doctor concurred. "I suppose it *could* be androgenic..."

"…but it doesn't look like typical PCOS-type, does it?" Mr Bowtie said. "Rather *odd*."

The two agreed that, for now, there was little that could be done other than to watch and wait.

"It's not that bad at the moment," Bowtie turned round to tell me, leaving no room for debate. "But if it does get worse in the coming months, then you can come back. We'll give you a prescription for a wig or something."

The mornings where I couldn't face looking at my reflection, the evenings where I'd forensically check tagged Facebook photos for my shiny scalp peeking through the glare of disco lights, those weekends spent visiting hair clinics and calculating whether my student budget would stretch to hair weaving systems – none of it was needed, right? Because if a dermatologist said my hair loss wasn't that bad, then I must have been over-reacting. Maybe I needed to stop being so vain.

I was turfed out of the appointment room with a paper handout explaining a hormone-related hair loss called androgenic alopecia, even though that definitely, possibly, probably, wasn't the cause of my hair loss. There was no arranged follow-up, no offer of counselling, and no acknowledgement of the fact that I was only *just* old enough to be out of children's services.

Far from having a concrete answer and definitive next steps, as I wandered out of the Victorian-era hospital, I was left with a distinct lack of hope. And that lack of hope is the most depressing outcome of all.

With hindsight, the initial 'diffuse thinning' stage of hair loss that I experienced in those early years was likely due to a mixture of lupus and having a cirrhotic liver (my diagnosis of PCOS was removed…twelve years later). Little did I know that, in just under a year of that dermatology appointment, a powered-up version of alopecia would commence after I started medication to dampen my immune system which was going crazy thanks to AIH.

This second time round, the hair loss was quite literally on steroids. Frizzy clumps of tumbleweed began to fall out everywhere: on my clothes, in my food, between the pages of laboratory books. If I ran my hand through my hair, threads upon threads would fall out, as if they were competing to parachute out of the follicles the fastest, entangling themselves between my fingers on their way.

I quickly figured that the best way to keep my remaining hair was to simply stop touching it and washing it. Shampooing only once a week caused it to morph into a greasy mop, like an illuminated arrow pointing out quite how threadbare my hair really was. The longer I left it unwashed, the more easily it tangled up into one big, rat-tailed, knotted birds' nest.

Every morning, I'd wake up an hour earlier just to wage war

against my reflection, positioning my barnet such that no bald spot could peek through. I'd sprinkle abrasive hair fibres and spritz cheap brown dry shampoo a little too liberally on the roots, desperately hoping that these amateur tactics would go some way to thickening what remained of my hair. All they did was dye my pillowcases a hint of brown.

Even walking through Primark's hair accessories section was somewhat triggering. I'd dream of wearing one of their decorative pearl headbands or, ye gods, a velvet scrunchie. Instead, I was relegated to a daily artful arrangement of approximately 43 functional hairpins, each one purposefully securing a thin section of limp hair-hay such that nothing would move accidentally from the impact of a slight breeze, revealing the true extent of the thinness. Defying the laws of physics, the hairpins somehow worked to create volume.

Within six months of starting steroids, my hair had lost most of its density. I was unable to fashion it into anything other than an ever-shrinking bun, and venturing outside on windy days was a no-no in case my hair blew the wrong way. A forecast of rain would bring with it a precipitation of panic; I refused to leave the house unless necessary, lest the dampness pasted my hair down flat against my skull and split into sections of lanky ravines like a sewer rat that had fallen on hard times. If you've ever visited Edinburgh, you'll understand the aforementioned weather criteria meant I couldn't leave the house for three quarters of the year. And on the rare occasions that sunshine broke through, it became an enemy too; not only did the rays cast a glaring spotlight over the shininess of my scalp, but there also ran the risk of potential sunburn with a lack of natural protection.

Fed up with greasy hair, I switched up my strategy, washing it every day rather than never. This time the battle was against my hairdryer, as I tried to frizz up certain sections to give an illusion of depth. It was a recurring nightmare amidst the ongoing whirlwind of my new medicalised life.

I'd wake up and bathe in a blissful microsecond where I'd forget that I had been diagnosed with irreversible liver disease and that my hair was a perennial shitshow, but consciousness would gradually kick in and bring with it the gut-wrenching realisation that my life was, indeed, a complete omnishambles. I'd then slowly – and gently, so as not to facilitate any more damage – lift my head and inspect the pillow for overnight casualties. Short of fastening yourself into a straitjacket, it's really difficult to restrict movement during sleep, so I made do with praying that I hadn't moved my head too much to disturb what little hair clung on.

The cruellest gut punch of alopecia is that, whereas at the start I'd fear the huge clumps of hair scattered over my pillow in the morning, the loss gradually lessened over time. Not because the rate of loss was slowing down, or reversing, but because I simply had less hair to lose.

At no point did I consider going back to the dermatology clinic. Whilst I expressed my distress to a GP about losing my hair, I didn't want to risk having to face that bowtie again. I'd probably be told it *still* wasn't bad enough.

Other doctors did try to make things better, at least notionally. I was cc'd onto a clinic letter where a consultant had ordered some more hormonal tests to, and I quote, "get to the root of the problem". But the overwhelming sentiment slowly dawned on me: in amongst the melee of my other medical problems, hair loss wasn't going to kill me. I needed to prioritise getting the deadly stuff under control.

That perspective, whilst realistic and sensible, did the square root of nothing to ease the fact that hair loss is inherently and debilitatingly stressful. It's a loss of control. It's the not knowing how long it's going to take to sort out a presentable hairstyle each morning. It's the loss of feeling – *whisper it* – attractive. It's the realisation that nobody knows at what stage this will end. In complete baldness? With the loss of eyebrows and eyelashes, too?

It's not knowing how fast this will happen, or why it's happening in the first place. The unknowns. The loneliness. The direct comparisons I still make, not necessarily to celebrities with their enviably glossy and unobtainable, perfect hair, but more to *normal* people in *normal* life who have *normal* hair. Hair loss was a visible marker of how I'd been shunted onto a dysfunctional runaway train track. Trying to rationalise the situation, I would remind myself that, really, I never had control of what my hair was like in the first place. But rationalising does little to stop the grief.

Googling 'hair loss' in bleak moments of doomsday thinking left me reading hundreds of upsetting accounts of ladies in their menopausal era suffering with thinning or receding hairlines. Patricia, 56, was struggling to come to terms with a "loss of her femininity", whereas Mandy, 64, worried about whether her husband of 30 years would still "find her attractive" without her golden tresses. And whilst I felt sorry for these women, I would find a not-insignificant part of me lacing my empathy with a twisted bitterness. That part of me thought that women who were going through this at a later stage of life had already had their time in the sun, their youth, their season of vitality and fertility. Outside of cancer patients, there seemed to be a distinct lack of younger ladies facing hair loss. I had only just got rid of the acne that blighted most of my teens[31] and hadn't even fully launched myself off nature's starting blocks. It felt more than a wee bit *unfair*.

Yet in the glimpses when I would ease up on feeling sorry for myself, I would defect straight over to feeling guilty about feeling upset. I deemed myself pathetic for caring about hair when I should have been grateful to even be alive. *You're not facing something terminal, Kirsty,* I'd sometimes tell myself. *Get a grip.*

But I could never fully buy into having such a stiff upper lip. Because here's the thing: it's unfair to lose your hair if you're 19, or if you're 49, or if you're 90. It's upsetting regardless of whether you're a woman, man, child, or someone in between. Yet male hair loss can be the butt of a joke – we've all seen the memes of flights to Turkey rammed full of men with shaved crowns – and it's not socially tabooed. Hell, it's even lauded as a sign of high testosterone count and virility.

*Female* baldness, on the other hand, seems to be shrouded in much more emotional complexity. We (and I refer to 'we' as women, here) don't tend to talk openly about female hair loss, despite it being relatively common at different stages of a woman's life, from pregnancy through to menopause. Why? Is it because we fear it, and to not talk of it almost works as a voodoo charm to stop it happening to us? Does our discomfort stem from a reluctance to admit that women are judged far more harshly on their appearances? That their intrinsic sense of worth sometimes depreciates in line with their deviation from what is socially accepted as 'pretty' – that they are 'less' of a person without a healthy head of hair? And who is doing the judging? Men? (Name me a man who notices

---

31 When I say *blighted*, it's not an exaggeration: it still stings to think of the time I was called 'pepperoni pizza face' by some kids going into school one day.

a changed haircut.) Is it, then, our fear of judgement from other women? Or worse, from ourselves?

My hair never grew back to its original thickness, and I now wear wigs. Now, I *know* it's superficial to bemoan a lack of attractiveness, but when I see my threadbare hair in the mirror, I'm still a little disappointed. Physical beauty is both fleeting and subjective, but that doesn't make it any less gutting to feel that I haven't lived out my 'prettiness' to its full potential. There have been times since losing my hair when I've felt pretty, but it's been the output of a calculated illusion. It's fake: a wig and makeup. It's not even a case of faking it until I make it, it's faking it until I can fake it really well. I do not feel – and truly have never felt – 'pretty' without a wig on. I look ill.

Hair loss is an all-encompassing loss. It can feel like a loss of one's identity, of one's confidence, of one's ability to go out and live life. It's a loss of recognising the face in the mirror, the version of ourselves which we present to the world. It's a loss of something which you take for granted. It's a loss of the naivety that accompanies an illness-free life. It's not just hair falling out. It's so, so much more.

## ...AND ON WIGS

With the same incredulity as the Singaporean hairdresser when I showed him Emma Watson as my hair inspiration, I eyed the mound of plastic curls attached to a netted weave lying on the bedside table. I then looked up at Mum, and back down again at the wig. In her depths of desperation, unable to listen to me sobbing down the phone every evening from my student flat, she had turned to sieving through Amazon's wig selection to find one that vaguely resembled my natural hair.

"I think it's very –" she began a little hesitantly, "– realistic. Very *you*." By this stage, a little over a year of starting steroid medication, I would quite happily have settled for a renaissance of the Singaporean frizz pyramid if it meant that I could wear my hair down without a huge bald patch showing.

Unwrapping the wig from its plastic sheath, I watched as the curls released themselves and sprung to life, before slipping it on awkwardly over my scalp. A distinctly plastic aroma wafted around as I sidled over on the bed in front of the mirror. My heart, so full of expectation, so optimistic that this £30 contraption would solve all my problems, plummeted as I saw what can only be described as my metamorphosis into a slightly chubby member of Michael Flatley's Riverdance troupe.

"What do you reckon?" Mum's eyes, pleading for a positive reaction, met with mine in the mirror. I turned wordlessly to face her, before plunging backwards onto my childhood bed and planting a pillow firmly over my face.

"I just want my old life back, Mum," I cried into the pillow, struggling to regulate my breathing in between muffled sobs that felt like they originated from the very pit of my stomach. To paraphrase Joni Mitchell, I didn't know what I had, 'til the thick Hagrid curls of my teenaged years were gone.

After that Amazon wig was relegated to the back of a cupboard, I set off to what felt like last chance saloon: a hair centre that specialised in 'toppers'. Whilst it might sound like something Fatboy Slim might have taken at a warehouse rave in the 90s, a topper is a half-wig that clips in to cover the top of your head, but leaves a portion of natural hair showing underneath. Toppers are the little siblings of 'full cap' wigs, where a whole head of hair is attached to fabric and popped on your head like a swimming cap.

The moment that topper clipped on, my shoulders unfurled from their default Quasimodo position. I inspected the sides and back of my head using a hand-mirror; the hair, styled in gentle waves, looked full, glossy and healthy. My face was framed. There was the tiniest spark of the version of myself I had lost, and I now had a tool with which to temporarily forget about the reality of my illness. I quite literally bounced out of the salon, stealing glances at myself in every window.

Despite this newfound confidence, I told nobody except my family, closest friends, and my then-boyfriend about my topper. As I was relocating for a new job around the same time, I just hoped that anyone I would meet would simply accept it as my real hair. Which they did, of course, because the only person who concentrates *that* hard on your appearance is, thankfully, you.

Mum agreed that the topper was a considerable upgrade from the Flatley-esque monstrosity. With a hint of déjà vu from the dermatology appointment, my boyfriend at the time said that, whilst my fake hair was "nice", he thought my natural birds' nest wasn't "that bad" in the first place. I decided to ignore his opinions and focus on how much more confident – not to mention warmer – wearing the hair made me. On reflection, I'm still not quite sure how I feel about his response, but I'll give him the benefit of the doubt because I think he was trying to be kind.

It's difficult to express how much of a lifesaver this topper was. It was quite possibly the best investment I have ever made, for it quickly became a brunette comfort blanket with which I could face the world. It eliminated the stress of the mornings spent fixing up my hairdo. It allowed me to wear those pretty headbands from Primark. Whilst I couldn't tie my hair up or go swimming or do rigorous exercise in it, and it frizzed up in humidity, it allowed me to feel like a 'normal' person again. And *that* was priceless.

A couple years later, however, I found that I no longer even had enough natural hair to adequately support the clips on the topper. The topper itself also began to look past its prime, so it was time to rev up a gear. Full-cap wigs sound like they would be an easy transition, but the problem is that they can be very…*extra.* Some of them look a bit too perfect, and it's easy for the wig to end up wearing the person, rather than the other way round. What's more, there is a mindboggling choice available. So much choice, in fact, that it's difficult to pick just one. Thing is, it's equally difficult to swap from long blonde curls on Monday to a ginger bob on Friday, without anyone noticing.

And so, aged 26, I decided if I wanted to enjoy the benefits of fake hair – having great hair within ten seconds flat – then I needed to really *own* wearing them. Having downed the confidence juice, I rocked up at work one morning wearing a mane of tumbling waves. The guts it takes to wear a wig cannot be underestimated; walking into that office was one of the most anxiety-inducing things I have done to date.

Whenever someone complimented me – and many people did, with one colleague kindly saying I resembled a 1950s movie star – I thanked them, before quickly following up with an admission that it wasn't real. Why not just say thank you and carry on? Firstly, people's reactions to wig reveals are priceless. But more seriously, it's because every single time I tell someone who's ever admired my hair that "it's actually a wig", whether that person is the lady serving coffees at the Hilton in Glasgow or the endoscopy nurse who's adjusting my oxygen tubes, I hope it chips away a tiny chunk of the stigma surrounding hair loss and wig-wearing.

Because whilst this stigma has arguably been reduced over the years (not just because of my efforts, obviously, but by a concerted societal move to be more accepting of visible differences), it still exists. Many hairdressing salons continue to chauffeur clients with alopecia down back-alley staircases into basement rooms to try on wigs. And whilst a huge number of film and television celebrities (both male and female) wear wigs, us mere mortals are left to assume that it's all achievable with the right gels and savvy use of a Dyson Airwrap. Spoiler alert: it's not.

When I began to feel at relative ease wearing full wigs, it suddenly had the potential to be great fun. The freedom to switch between pink, ginger and brunette within an hour is liberating. I can be bobbed or long, curly or sleek, with bangs or a side part; ultimately, I need never have a bad hair day again. I have razor-sharp bobs with which I feel businesslike, ombre waves that allow me to channel my Sienna Miller-boho-circa-2004 vibes, and wigs that I plait in the style of a minor character in *Game of Thrones* before putting them on my head.

When I was 15 and as shallow as a puddle, I'd imagine myself living the life of a career high-flyer in London by my mid-20s. I'd have it all sorted out by then: the cellulite on my knees would be gone, and I'd have figured out some way to slim my cankles. My wardrobe would consist of Reiss dresses in jewel colours, and the icing on the cake would be having my hair coiffed to perfection. Oh, how I misjudged *so* many aspects. But I like to think that, in a roundabout way, I've got the hair bit down to a tee.

Sure, there are times when I don't feel comfortable wearing a wig. Often, I'll see a photo of myself in one of my cheaper wigs with a fringe and have deep retrospective cringe, because it looks fake, and I look silly. Every single night, after that day's wig has been taken off, I wish more than anything that I had my old hair back. I long to be able to scrape my old curls up into a messy bun, or to choose holiday destinations without considering whether it'll be too hot to wear fake hair. Oh, to have MRI scans without the indignity of whipping off a wig (and its metallic clips) in front of the radiology team, or to visit the seaside and not constantly monitor the swooping seagulls lest one of them poos on my barnet (this has happened before, and I had to throw the wig out).

Sometimes I often wonder if, by wearing wigs, I'm not confronting the reality of my situation. In a basic sense, I'm still hiding, still covering up. Should I focus my efforts on building up the confidence to say, '*fuck it*', and walk out my house with threadbare hair? Perhaps. As I get older, I find myself being more comfortable with going to Sainsbury's, or swimming, or to the gym, with my hair *au naturelle*. But am I a traitor to the feminist cause by giving in to societal expectations of having a glossy mane? I don't think so.

If I didn't have my wigs, then I probably wouldn't have been able to get a job. I wouldn't have the confidence to put myself forward, to be taken seriously in almost all the things I do. Wigs have been the single most important anti-depressant in my life. They are my ride or die for dealing with my chronic illness, and I feel less comfortable without one. Whilst I have the utmost admiration for ladies who rock the thinning/bald look (many do, and look amazing), I personally don't feel my best that way.

I like to look nice, because it makes me feel nice, and I deserve to feel attractive, like any other person. Have I felt attractive whilst wearing a wig? Yes. Have I felt insecure whilst wearing a wig? Also yes. Does the world end when your hair falls out? Is Fleabag right – is hair everything? Of course not.

The crux lies in understanding that wigs empower me. Hair loss might be outside my sphere of influence, but wigs provide me with the choice to respond in a way that I *can* control. Life's too short to not feel good, so if you don't mind, please pass me that head of hair. Just *not* the Riverdance one.

# ON HOW THE LIVER WORKS…

We're a few chapters in, so I'm assuming you're willing to join me further on this ride through medical malarky. If so, then buckle up, because we're now propelling ourselves towards some pretty dense stuff.

Firstly, though, I want you to do a couple of exercises whilst you're reading this. (Nothing strenuous, don't worry.) Take a deep breath in through your nose. Hold it for a couple seconds. Now let that beautiful breath tumble back out through your mouth. Look away from the page briefly, close your eyes and just wallow in that nothingness. Hopefully that feels good.

Next action: have a think about what you've eaten today. Maybe some porridge, a cheeky midday cuppa. You might have pushed that boat right out and had a fish supper. Think about that food being digested right now, all those calories burning up to provide energy for you to do stuff. Magical, isn't it? That portion of chips is now letting you read these words, whilst breathing, whilst pushing blood round your veins, whilst keeping your temperature in check. Not too shabby for some chips. Wherever you are, pause. Take stock of your body for letting you just…*be*.

When I was studying chemistry at university, none of my experiments in the laboratory panned out as the textbooks said they would. If the assignment was to make a cobalt blue powder, I would invariably end up crystallising a greyish mush with orange flecks. One student[32] made a mini catalytic converter in the lab that exploded and set off a fire alarm requiring the attendance of most of Edinburgh City's fire department, yet somehow that prototype works seamlessly every day in cars across the world. The take-home message from my degree was that science somehow pulls it all together for us in real life.

Applying this maxim to human medicine, it's just as well it all works in real life. Considering how many processes could go wrong within the body, never mind the array of external invaders ready to wreak havoc, it's quite honestly baffling that anyone can make it through the day without their toes spontaneously erupting in gangrenous pain.

*Your body*, to quote the morally-questionable-but-admittedly-good-guitarist John Mayer, *is a wonderland.* I daresay this wasn't quite the direction he was pitching for with those lyrics (the rest of the song is a tad risqué) but from a medical perspective, every single person on this planet is a wee biological miracle.

If John Mayer was to rerecord his song in a parallel universe, and make it specific to my body, he might be tempted to change the lyrics of *Your Body is a Wonderland* to reference a *Slightly Toxic Wasteland.* But at the end of the day, it's the only

---

[32] Not me.

wasteland I'll ever get to live in. I know its map, I'm prepared for its freakish weather systems, and I've grown to see the appeal in its quirks. Perhaps living in a wonderland is a little overrated anyways, for can it ever be appreciated without having the experience of things going wrong for comparison?

## An Office of Organs

Wonderland or wasteland, the human body is an amazing place. If we anthropomorphise five of its vital organs into office workers, it's easy to visualise the **brain** as being the experienced but cocky CEO powerhouse of the firm. It's the narcissist who calls the big shots…and knows it. If the brain leaves, then the whole company loses direction damn quickly, and its share price flounders overnight.

The **heart,** meanwhile, joined fresh out of uni on the graduate programme and has speedily made its way to the upper echelons, with its eye on a role in senior management. It aces performance reviews, networks well, and does a steady amount of work, day in and day out.

The **kidneys** are the two extremely competent but socially awkward colleagues who thrive on working in the gloomy bowels of the office. They spend their days endlessly sanitising the less favourable company data before it leaks to the public. If one of them quit, the other would be miserable without their only work buddy, and be overworked, but would stick it out because they can't be arsed applying for another job.

The **lungs** are the chillaxed and knowledgeable, but somewhat reticent, colleagues who have been at the company for decades, know the role inside out, and can deal with a lot of strain when required to firefight any dramas. They work closely with the heart, having taken it under their wing during the graduate scheme, but think the heart works too hard for the salary.

And then we have the **liver**: the eternal people-pleaser, the one who stoically spins too many plates and does such a good job at keeping them all going that nobody else fully realises quite how much work it's doing. The liver runs the bake sales and organises the meal selection spreadsheet for team Christmas dinners, in addition to firing out emails well after midnight and joining 6am conferences after a spin class, imprinting a tiny bit of itself in every single department to the extent that it becomes indispensable. The liver also organises the CEO's diary, so if the liver takes a day off (although it never really does, having downloaded the Teams app to its personal phone and therefore being permanently available), then the brain hasn't got a clue what's going on.

The liver is the only organ in the office who can detoxify an Excel spreadsheet using *VLOOKUP* without needing to launch a YouTube tutorial. Soon enough, the liver becomes known as the Excel Expert, which it gets a bit miffed at, because there are over 500 other equally important jobs it does that seem to get no recognition. Other employees take advantage of having an Excel Expert to hand, putting way too many columns on their Excels, causing rendering issues and calculating errors. Yet every time their spreadsheet goes non-responsive with the scrolling wheel of doom, they laugh it off with a cavalier guffaw.

"Oh, God help the liver try to fix *this* mess!"

Over time, the liver gets tired but would never refuse to help, so it keeps on doing everything. But then other stuff happens in the liver's life – say its dog dies, and then it gets a speeding ticket – and it all becomes too much for the liver to handle. The plates it's been spinning start to spin more slowly at first…and then come crashing to the ground. The corporation grinds to a halt because, as the liver is now so intrinsically involved in everyone's processes, nobody can do their jobs without it.

It doesn't take a genius to work out the metaphor I'm pitching for here. The liver does *way* more than detoxifying the alcohol after a boozy night out.

## The Anatomy Bit

As a top-tier liver fangirl, I think it is only right that we do a high-level overview of the organ's amazing anatomy.

The liver is the **largest internal organ** (the skin being the biggest organ overall, by size) and **weighs between 1.3 kg and 1.8 kg**[iii] in an average person. If we're properly technical, the liver is tucked up cosily in the right 'hypochondrium' of the body and extends out into the left 'hypochondrium'.[iv] Think of your liver as a spongy wedge around the size of a rugby ball that starts under your right boob and moves across your abdomen to behind your left one.

Generally, any living thing with a spinal cord also has a liver[v] – so that covers all vertebrates, from stingrays to spaniels. Human livers have **two key sources of blood**[vi]:

1. The **hepatic artery** (containing 25% of the liver's blood supply) provides oxygenated blood to the liver straight from the heart, and
2. The **hepatic portal vein** (doing the bulk of the heavy lifting with the remaining 75% of the supply[vii]) provides the liver with partially de-oxygenated blood that is rich with nutrients (that have been absorbed by the small intestine) from the gastrointestinal tract,

gallbladder, pancreas, and spleen.[33]

Blood flows back out of the liver, too. Blood drains through hepatic veins in the liver to a super big vein called the **inferior vena cava.** This is the largest vein in the body and takes blood to the heart.[viii] The key takeaway here is that there's **a lot of blood going in and out of your liver.** In fact, roughly 13% of the total amount of blood in your body at any given moment in time will be in or around the liver system.[ix] It filters about 1.5 litres of the red stuff every minute of every day[x], separating out any harmful substances and processing beneficial nutrients and chemicals, which is the reason why it's so important that the liver tissue stays soft and healthy to allow all this blood to flow through. When liver tissue gets damaged for whatever reason, it becomes quite tough. This makes it harder for the blood to pass through, which can then be dangerous.

The liver is split into anatomical sections, called **lobes.**[xi] These lobes contain thousands of **lobules**, which can be thought of as mini lobes. Each lobule – and remember, there are *thousands* of these bad boys – is shaped like a little hexagon. (Whilst I'm not religious, I can't help but wonder at the beauty of design in nature.) A lobule is essentially a structural unit of the liver which contains lots of **hepatocytes** – a fancy name for liver cells.[xii] Don't worry if I've lost you (I've lost myself somewhere in this paragraph, too); the headliner here is that the **liver contains lots and lots of liver cells.**

The liver, along with its blood vessels, is nicely wrapped up in a pretty layer of loose tissue known as **Glisson's Capsule**.

---

[33] Think of the spleen as your personal blood guru, the gallbladder as the thing that stores bile which helps digest your food, and the pancreas as the control panel for your blood sugar levels. Your GI (gastrointestinal) tract is, put simply, the route that food travels from your mouth through to your backside.

I mention this specifically as a shout-out to its namesake, Francis Glisson. Glisson was the original mature student, who not only had the most banging haircut[34] of the 1600s but also graduated in medicine aged 37 and became one of the founders of the Royal Society.[xiii] He achieved all this whilst also doing a lot of important work to determine the anatomy of the liver.

## What does the liver actually do?

The liver is not just a pretty face. Everything we ingest gets digested by the stomach and intestine, and then absorbed into the blood. This nutrient-rich blood then leaves the intestines and makes its way through the liver. If the body was a nightclub, the liver is a bit like the bouncer who **weeds out the harmful toxins** (such as alcohol, drugs and pollutants) and converts these into less dangerous products. At the same time, the liver **ensures the body receives the nutrients it needs**, extracting the good stuff from the blood and making these nutrients available for use in the body either immediately, or when needed in future. For example, the liver extracts sugar (glucose) from the blood and stores it under the alias of glycogen, which is then converted back to glucose when required to **provide energy for our bodies.**[xiv] The liver also acts like a hotel where iron, copper and vitamins (A, D, E, K, B12) chill out for future use when the body needs them.[xv]

The liver, being the absolute powerhouse that it is, creates a product called **bile**[xvi], a yellow-orangey fluid which helps to break down and absorb fats from food (thereby helping them to be absorbed by the body). When waste products have been broken down by the liver into non-harmful substances, the products are disposed of either into the bile or into the blood.

[34] Google it, it beats anything that I got in a Singapore hair salon

Bile by-products enter the intestines and depart the body in your poo, whereas blood by-products are filtered out by the kidneys and leave the body in the form of pee. Clever, eh?

The liver is responsible for producing hormones which **regulate blood pressure** and **aid cell growth and development**. The liver also helps with the generation of amino acids which then join together to make proteins, which ultimately help to **build and repair muscles and bones**, and can be an energy source. Furthermore, the liver clears up a substance called bilirubin, which is a by-product of the breakdown of red blood cells. If the liver doesn't do this, the bilirubin starts building up and turns the skin and eyes a Bart Simpson-yellow, which is called **jaundice**.

The liver also produces blood clotting factors (to help promote **wound healing** and **avoiding excessive bleeding**) and specific proteins including albumin, which helps to carry **hormones, vitamins and enzymes** around the body. The liver **gets rid of bacteria from the blood** using something called Kupffer cells, which sound more at home in a Tom Cruise film, but nonetheless work by encapsulating bad-guy bacteria and viruses and excreting them from the bloodstream.[xvii]

As if that's not enough, the liver also **produces heat** through a process called thermogenesis, which helps to maintain a steady body temperature. When the body's temperature drops, the liver will release some glucose into the bloodstream. This glucose will then be used by cells to produce energy, which also creates heat. This raises the body's temperature and prevents hypothermia.[xviii]

I hereby conclude our biology lesson (and no, there is no exam after reading this).

# …AND WHAT HAPPENS WHEN IT DOESN'T

I'll say it again for those at the back: a healthy liver is essential for the routine functioning of a human body. Unfortunately, there are also a mind-boggling number of ways in which all these miraculous hepatic processes can go wrong, often causing inflammation of the liver tissue. This inflammation is called **hepatitis (*hep-ah-tie-tiss*)**. Whilst a sizeable portion of the public connect liver damage exclusively to alcohol or drug misuse, there are over 100 causes of liver disease.[xix]

## What happens when the liver gets damaged?

Luckily, the liver is a fairly stoic organ; it can often withstand a fair amount of damage before it stops working altogether. But therein lies its (quite literally) fatal flaw: damaged livers sometimes remain broadly asymptomatic until the very end stages of the disease, meaning that the last-chance-saloon of liver failure can rear its head out of the blue. If your liver fails, it's game over for the rest of your body.

Whilst we have dialysis to help failing kidneys, artificial pumps for broken hearts, and ventilation devices for struggling lungs, there's no 'get out of jail free' card for a failing liver.

The level of damage to the liver tissue can be simplistically considered as a sliding scale. If the cause of hepatitis is not stopped in good time, then the liver tissue initially reaches a stage called **fibrosis (*fiy-bro-siss*)**. Fibrosis is early scarring of the liver tissue, when the tissue becomes less healthy, and the liver can't cope as well as it used to. Sometimes a fibrotic liver can prove symptomatic, with patients experiencing a general sense of being unwell, fatigue, itchy skin, sore tummy, loss of appetite, feeling sick and/or muscle pain.[xx]

If the damage is stopped at this point, then the fibrosis can be 'healed', back to being healthy liver tissue. This is thanks to the liver being the only organ that can regenerate after damage. Nine times out of ten, when I have told people that I have a bad liver, they've responded with a look of horror that melts quickly into compassionate relief when the lightbulb flashes on in their head.

"Oh, but, but…the liver regenerates, right? You'll be ok, right?"

Wrong. Like many urban myths, there's an *element* of truth in this assumption, but it's only a half-truth. The liver's regeneration mechanism isn't well understood, but we do know that if 90% of the liver volume was removed, then the 10% that was left would be able to regenerate into a full-sized liver.[xxi] However, the liver doesn't regenerate in the miraculous way we are told it does, like a magical organ salamander; it can only regenerate to a certain degree.[xxii]

If the cause of damage is not stopped in time, the fibrosis

can slowly turn into an end-stage, irreversible form of liver damage, called **cirrhosis (*sir-oh-siss*)**. If the liver is cirrhotic, there is no way on Earth that liver is going to be regenerating itself like a phoenix. Cirrhotic livers are less able to do their jobs effectively, but even within the category of cirrhosis, patients can have varying levels of disease.

**Compensated cirrhosis,** as the name suggests, means that to all intents and purposes, the liver is scarred but still manages to get on with the day job. This category is where I currently reside (and I'd like to keep it this way for as long as I can). I'd prefer to be compensated with a penthouse flat in New York, or a waistline like Shakira, but that's life. Compensated cirrhosis, however, does not mean *unaffected* by cirrhosis.

I tire very easily, especially with exercise, and am always slightly anaemic[35]. A day out will either require a nap halfway, or a couple days' recovery afterwards. My entire body is littered with bruises due to low platelets. My nails are brittle, and my skin sometimes gets itchy at night. Occasionally, I'll wake up with terrible leg cramps, or alternatively a sharp, stitch-like pain in my upper right side that takes my breath away. I am ruled out of taking a range of medication (certain antibiotics, most contraceptives, and anti-depressants) because my liver is too poorly to metabolise them effectively. I have increased blood pressure ('portal hypertension') in one of the main veins in the liver which means that I'm at risk of spontaneous and potentially fatal internal bleeding. This, in turn, requires checking with endoscopies every few months.

I am also at an increased risk of liver cancer, requiring an ultrasound scan twice a year to check for abnormalities. There

---

[35] Anaemia is when your body doesn't have enough red blood cells to get oxygen to the tissues.

are spider veins on my face, hands and all over my legs. My hair still falls out, and I still do not get periods (which means, due to my womb lining not shedding, I'm also at increased risk of womb cancer, unless I have an IUD). I don't clear infections easily and as such they can progress into more serious infections very quickly. Any time I have a fever or sore throat, I need to organise blood tests pronto. Otherwise, my blood will be checked on a frequency ranging between every couple of months to once a week (or daily, if staying in hospital).

I can't eat too many salty or fatty foods, and sometimes I'm just not hungry at all. My bowels are more unpredictable than Donald Trump and I have little pockets of fluid in my abdomen which run the risk of becoming infected. I get quite shaky sometimes. I can't play contact sports in case my spleen, which is very large, explodes (not the correct medical term). I get hot flushes, but need a hot water bottle taped against me whilst working from home because my circulation is sluggish.

That's the liver damage alone, when everything is otherwise relatively stable. During a flare of my AIH, all these symptoms can become amplified. And *then* there's all the side effects from medication, which we'll cover later.

I don't intend for this to be a 'woe is me' diatribe; I'm merely pointing out what can happen when your liver still technically functions, but isn't in tip-top condition. The scary thing is, you'd probably never know all this was going on from looking at me.

**Decompensated cirrhosis** is when the liver can no longer function. This is when the alarm bells really start ringing. It's equivalent to that bit in the Titanic film where the engine room gets blasted to bits with water bursting through. Rose and Jack are tapping their SOSs on the lead piping, and the whole ship goes belly up.

Decompensated cirrhosis brings with it life-threatening complications.[xxiii] One of these includes a condition called **ascites (*ahh-sigh-teez*),** where a substantial amount of fluid leaks into the abdominal cavity. This causes patients to have painfully distended bellies, and requires draining or diuretic medication to avoid infection. Decompensated cirrhosis brings with it a greatly increased risk of variceal bleeding due to portal hypertension. Portal hypertension also puts extra strain on vessels taking blood to the kidneys, and can result in **kidney failure**.[xxiv]

**Jaundice** (yellowing of the skin and eyes) can occur when the liver can no longer clear bilirubin sufficiently well.[xxv] As if all this wasn't enough, the brain can be affected by decompensated cirrhosis, too. When the liver is unable to filter out toxins, ammonia can accumulate in the bloodstream. This can lead to neurological dysfunction[xxvi] in the form of what is referred to as **encephalopathy (*en-seff-ah-lop-ah-thee*)**. If not treated in sufficient time, hepatic encephalopathy can cause personality changes, confusion, coma and ultimately death.

The line between compensated and decompensated cirrhosis can be very thin; I've had periods of decompensation (for example, having ascites and an internal bleed), but recovered back to a compensated state. More often, the only treatment for decompensated cirrhosis is a liver transplant.

## What Can Cause Liver Damage?

*Viral hepatitis*

Hepatitis can be caused through contracting a virus.

**Hepatitis A, B, C, D[36] and E** are viruses that can be contracted through a variety of modes including drinking contaminated water, eating improperly cooked meats or unwashed fruits, or through contact with contaminated bodily fluid (via childbirth, sharing razors or toothbrushes, needlestick injury, contaminated blood transfusions, or intravenous drug use).[xxvii]

If this rings a bell, it might be because you'll have heard of the blood donation scandal, whereby many people contracted hepatitis C after having infected blood donations between 1970 and the 1990s. An estimated 30,000 people in the UK were mistakenly given blood products that contained either HIV or hepatitis C.[xxviii] The doctors didn't realise until it was too late, when many patients had developed liver cirrhosis and ultimately required liver transplants or passed away. Today, blood donations are screened for hepatitis viruses, so this error shouldn't happen again.

There are now vaccines available for hepatitis A, B (the vaccine for hepatitis B also protects against hepatitis D) and E, but currently no vaccine exists for hepatitis C.[xxix]

*Fatty liver disease (also known as MASLD or NAFLD)*

Lifestyle choices can play a role in liver damage, too. **Fatty liver disease** is (no surprises here) a condition where there is too much fat in the liver. It's linked to a rise in obesity rates. It is estimated that 1 in 5 people in the UK has some form of fatty liver disease.[xxx]

Contributing factors include type 2 diabetes, a sedentary

---

[36] D is a wee bit of a special case, because you can only get hepatitis D if you already have hepatitis B.

lifestyle, too many sugary and fatty foods in the diet, and being overweight. Fatty deposits in the liver can result, over time, in mild to moderate fibrosis. The fibrosis, if left untreated, can then progress to cirrhosis. Steps like eating less unhealthy food and increasing exercise levels should improve the fatty liver condition in the earlier stages of the disease, avoiding further damage.[xxxi]

*Autoimmune disorders*

Sometimes, lifestyle and diet do not play a role in the development of liver damage, and instead, the enemy lies within. In my own series of unfortunate events, my immune system decided that it is not busy enough with fighting off foreign invaders and started attacking my liver cells instead. My condition is called **autoimmune hepatitis (AIH)**, but there are other autoimmune conditions wherein the liver is damaged in a slightly different way.

**Primary biliary cholangitis (PBC)** involves the immune system attacking the bile ducts (the tubes that transport bile to the intestine) within the liver. This, in turn, means that bile can't be cleared from the liver properly, and it begins to damage the liver tissue. Again, the trigger for this is so far unidentified, but the condition is more common in women.[xxxii]

Similarly, but not exactly the same, **primary sclerosing cholangitis (PSC)** is a chronic liver disease in which the bile ducts both inside *and outside* the liver become inflamed, scarred and eventually narrowed or blocked. Again, this causes bile to back up in the liver, causing damage. PSC is more common in men, and has a strong link with inflammatory bowel disease (IBD).[xxxiii]

*Congenital conditions*

Sometimes, people are born with conditions which means their livers are a little funky. **Biliary atresia**, for example, is a condition wherein the bile ducts don't develop normally in the womb, or become damaged soon after birth. It's not fully understood why this happens, other than a predisposition of a specific gene coupled with environmental factors (which is medical shorthand for *sorry, mate, we haven't got a clue*).[xxxiv]

The condition often initially appears to be indistinguishable from common neonatal jaundice (a harmless condition in otherwise healthy babies) but before long, infants with biliary atresia will develop other symptoms of a failing liver, including pale poo and dark urine. They may also fail to gain weight due to an inability to absorb vitamins.

Over time, the liver may develop cirrhosis and so babies with biliary atresia will require surgery (called the Kasai procedure) before they are two months old to remove the blockage in their bile ducts. This surgery creates a new passageway for bile to drain straight from their liver to their intestines, slowing down the rate of liver damage and delaying the need for transplant. Nonetheless, many patients with biliary atresia will require multiple liver transplants later in life.

**Wilson's disease** is another genetic condition whereby copper levels build up in several organs, including the liver. Normally the liver will remove excess copper from the body using bile, but this doesn't happen in people with Wilson's disease. This can lead to cirrhosis.[xxxv]

**Cystic fibrosis** patients might suffer from liver complications due to mucus build up in the bile ducts. Whilst this is rare, it can cause permanent liver damage and require a liver transplant.[xxxvi]

**Hereditary haemochromatosis** (bit of a tongue twister, that one) is another inherited condition whereby there is a predisposition by the liver to absorb too much iron. Over time, this can cause liver damage.[xxxvii]

*Other rare conditions*

There are other rare conditions which can cause liver damage, too. **Budd-Chiari Syndrome** involves problems with how the blood flows through the liver[xxxviii]. This leads to congestion and potential damage to the liver tissues.

Sometimes the cause of liver damage isn't known, even after investigations. This is called **cryptogenic cirrhosis.**

*Alcohol-related liver disease (ARLD)*

**ARLD** refers to liver damage caused by excessive alcohol intake. There are several stages of severity and a range of associated symptoms, but regrettably alcohol consumption is the leading cause of liver disease in the UK, accounting for 6 in 10 cases. It is estimated that up to 1 in 5 people in the UK drink alcohol in a way that could harm their liver.[xxxix]

## A Word on Liver Transplants

Regardless of the cause, the only treatment (and it is a treatment, not a cure) for end-stage liver disease is a liver transplant. So why not just give everyone with cirrhosis a liver transplant? Fair question. First things first, a liver transplant is massive abdominal surgery. It's not, as an ultrasound nurse once clumsily suggested to me, a matter of "whipping the bad liver out and putting a new one in" and waiting for the body to magically be as right as rain again.

With life-changing consequences in terms of physical and psychological recovery, and with the need for lifelong immunosuppression (though I'm already aboard this ship), a transplant is only considered if the patient is likely to survive the operation and has no other options. The risk of rejection (whereby the body's immune system cottons on that there's a massive foreign organ that's been put in place of the usual one) is high, even with anti-rejection drugs. It's even more of a risk in patients who already reject their own livers (a.k.a me). There are countless other risks throughout the remainder of a transplant recipient's life, alongside trying to ensure the original cause of the liver damage is addressed.

Moreover, there's not a plentiful supply of livers on ice, ready and waiting for everyone who needs one. Whilst 894[xl] people in the UK had a liver transplant between April 2024 and April 2025, there were still 616 people[xli] waiting on the liver transplant list (as of 31 March 2025). Some of these people will be waiting months, or even years, for a new liver, all the while suffering with some of those aforementioned symptoms of decompensated liver disease. Not every potential donor has organs suitable for transplantation. There are so many compatibility issues to overcome: family wishes, blood types, size, screening for different viruses which might nullify the ability to donate – all set against a backdrop of an ever-increasing demand pool with competing priorities.

To put it bluntly, liver transplantation is often the only alternative to death. Organ donation has the ability to completely transform a person's quality of life and provide years, if not decades, of health. It's an entirely personal decision, of course, but I would encourage you, my lovely reader, to consider your own decisions regarding organ donation. Personally, I believe that those who would readily accept an organ should also be willing to donate. Whilst the law in the UK is now on an opt-out basis, meaning everyone is elected *in* for donation unless they express wishes otherwise, the family of the deceased retain the right to refuse donation at the point of death.

This is why it's so important to ensure you have the conversation with your nearest and dearest. If you find it a difficult topic to bring out of nowhere, feel free to use this book as a segue. Thank you.

**How can we keep our livers healthy?**

Horrifyingly, there has been a **four-fold increase** in the number of deaths caused by liver disease in the UK over the last 50 years, and it is estimated that over 11,000 people die each year in the UK from liver damage. Now, I promised at the outset of this book that I wouldn't include any wellness lectures. That said, a staggering **90% of liver disease is preventable**[xlii], so I feel obliged to inform people of how to look after their livers.

It's arguably a lot easier said than done when considering wider socioeconomic issues of poverty and governmental alcohol/drug policy, but for most of us, the secret to keeping a healthy liver is as mundane as:

- Eating a balanced diet with lots of fruit and vegetables, wholegrains, and unprocessed food. You know the score. It's not rocket science. Eight slices of Victoria sponge for breakfast is not a liver-friendly diet.
- Maintaining a healthy weight and keeping active. Being obese puts your liver under strain and increases the risk

of fatty liver damage.

- Avoiding excessive alcohol intake. The NHS low-risk drinking guidance advises a maximum of 14 alcohol units per week (roughly six pints or six medium-sized glasses of wine) for both men and women. The crucial bit is that this week should also include three alcohol-free days, ideally in a row.[xliii]
- Protecting yourself against viral hepatitis. This includes following standard hygiene principles like not sharing razors or toothbrushes, practising basic food hygiene, using reputable tattoo parlours, having protected sex, and being vaccinated when travelling to regions with increased incidence of viral hepatitis.
- Stopping smoking. Smoking can make all types of liver disease worse, and can increase the risk of developing liver cancer.

It may be a boring message, but it's really important, so I will bang that drum like a Prohibition-era nun until I have no energy left in my bones. Liver disease is a silent killer. Love your liver, before it's too late.

# ON WHY ME-ISM

Occasionally, when producers are struggling for content on BBC Breakfast, they'll invite someone called Clive on with a health condition as part of a national awareness week. *Great,* I'll think, pouring milk into my cereal as I watch. *I'm all for raising awareness of different health problems. This is a great opportunity. Good on you, Clive.*

The presenters will ask Clive to explain how and when he was diagnosed, what medicines he takes, maybe even touch on how the condition affects his work or trips to the cinema every Thursday evening. There might, if they're really struggling to fill time, be a more probing question or two. Nothing too triggering, mind, for a Tuesday morning. There will be a video montage starting with his hospital pictures, emotional enough to have impact, but not tear-inducing. A family member, pet or close friend will be planted on the sofa next to him for moral support.

"Now, we happen to know that Clive here is most definitely what we'd call a strong character," the presenter will say, peering at their notes. "We've got it on good authority that you never complain or moan about your condition. You've never once asked '*why me?*', have you, Clive?"

Clive shrugs his shoulders a little, before straightening his back and puffing his chest out to show off his charity-branded t-shirt. "No, no, never. Not once. I just get on with it."

I'm really happy for people like Clive. Truly, I am. It's very noble to feel this way. After all, it's far better to crack on with life, making positive out of negative, rather than succumbing to a whirlpool of doom and never managing to swim back up. Right? Right.

Thing is, I find Clive's admission a wee bit hard to swallow down with my bowl of Crunchy Nut[37], because I struggle to believe that anyone who has been diagnosed with a serious, long-term, and therefore life-changing, condition would never ask *why the fuck* this had to happen to them.

In fact, I'm prepared to bet my bottom dollar that it's a sign of my sanity to howl at the moon at least once a month in an attempt to somehow better understand why – of all the billions of people on this planet – *I* have been specially selected to go through all this. I regularly consider what I might have done to upset the karma gods. Was it because I accidentally shoplifted a 'The Logical Song' CD from HMV in 2002 (I genuinely don't know how it fell into my bag, and I returned it when I realised)? Or because I didn't stand up for Rhiannon when the other kids put a black permanent marker dot on her cheek whilst she slept peacefully on the Belgium school trip?

I eat seven portions of veg a day and sponsor a guide dog

[37] I'm not a 24/7 angel when it comes to the healthy liver-friendly diet. Sometimes I go wild.

puppy. I'm generally a net-positive human. Of course, I don't do this exclusively in the hope that the universe shines favourably on me, but nonetheless, I often question why it doesn't add up. Despite learning fairly early on in life that being a good person does not guarantee an easy, healthy, fulfilling and pain-free ride, it never stops being galling to know that the inverse is true: the world is crammed full of people doing really shitty things without their comeuppance.

Why can't Cocaine Cassandra down the road deal with my health for a year? Why couldn't I just have *one* autoimmune problem, instead of two? Why couldn't I just have fibrosis of the liver, rather than already having the end-stage scarring?

Yet here I am, taking more than my fair share for the team, if we consider the team to be a nationwide statistical pool. I'm the one in 10,000[xliv] with AIH. The veneer of security in rarity is ripped off the moment you're diagnosed with a rare condition. No longer is there any sense of comfort upon hearing a healthcare professional say, "...but those symptoms are indicative of an incredibly *rare* condition, so chances are you *won't* have this".

The second you become a card-carrying member of the tiny group of people to whom the rarest of rare conditions has already graced their presence, the entry gates are prised open for a second, third or fourth knockout wave. The statistical reality is that, once a person has one set of serious health problems, the probability of becoming a magnet for others becomes higher. The logic of "I already have so much bad stuff, I can't possibly have any *more* things go wrong" applies less with each additional diagnosis or medication.

Whilst I sometimes try to tell myself that the 'why me' question is just as easily switched to 'well, why *not* me', the application of rationality doesn't lessen the blow of being in the firing line of unfairness. These conditions will be with me forever, and the chances are that my health will trend in an overall downwards trajectory. The most frustrating aspect is that nobody is at fault; it's pointless trying to attribute blame.

The key thing I've learned over the years is that sometimes I just need to wallow in that frustration. It's natural to be pissed off. It's okay to have moments where I feel resentful at the world, or to be jealous of the good health that others are blessed with, and spiteful of the lack of care with which they treat it. Hell, it's okay to eat the Crunchy Nut and not feel even a little bit guilty about it.

But whilst it's fine to know that it could be better, it's even more important to keep in mind that it could also be much worse. I know that some people might consider this attitude as 'toxic positivity', but I like to call it 'keeping things in perspective', because, really, often it *could* be a lot worse. Rather than spending too much time on wondering '*why me*', I try to reflect that frustrated energy back out more positively towards others, actively seeking out people or groups who have experienced or are experiencing difficult situations, and trying to help them. After all, most people experience their own 'why me' situation in one form or another.

I'm not trying to portray myself as some modern-day Lady Di, volunteering here, there and everywhere, but more simply stating that at times when I've been feeling really sorry for myself, I've found it incredibly helpful to switch the focus on to someone *other than me*. By homing in on that commonality between people, that shared sense of hardship, I've often been brought out of an insular mindset that can otherwise become a little overwhelming.

It is therefore disingenuous to paint "*why me*"-ism as an inherently negative trait. Perhaps a dose of *why-me*-ism can be healthy, if it follows through to positive outcomes such as gaining an awareness and acceptance of your disadvantages as a means of reflection and practising kindness towards others and, ultimately, oneself. I find it to be a way of reminding myself to be proud of how I continue living life as well as I can, despite these challenges.

Whilst I might be unlucky enough to be singled out for bad health-related things, there's a flipside: I might also be lucky enough to be singled out for good non-health-related things, too. I may well be the one in a million who has both lupus and AIH, but I could also be the one in a billion (don't quote me on the odds) who wins the lottery. Maybe I'm just an idiot who doesn't understand statistics, but it keeps me a little bit happier to think this way. Something bad is probably round the corner, but equally something good might be, too.

It will never be 'fair' that I was diagnosed with end-stage liver disease when I was young, but life never comes with a cast-iron guarantee against disparity. In fact, I'm beginning to think that it's all just one big corrupt casino filled with games of luck. Whilst I've been dealt a royal flush of rubbish health cards, they've been shuffled in with a lot of blessings, too. I reckon the two sides go hand in hand.

# ON SHIT HITTING THE PROVERBIAL FAN

*"It may seem hard to believe, but it's catastrophe that offers the most promise for an even richer life. This is the gateway to the good stuff. In other words, you never truly know which way the wind is blowing until the shit hits the fan."*

*Michael J. Fox*

Even if they're too cool to admit it, everyone loves a 90s tune. If there was a soundtrack to encapsulate my 2015, it would be Chumbawamba's Tubthumping remix (you know the one: *I get knocked down, but I get up again*). Until then, I had miraculously managed to duck under any Mike Tyson-strength blows of liver disease. All things considered, my liver had bravely kept doing its job, and the rest of my body begrudgingly played along. In the two years post-diagnosis, I had graduated, got a job, volunteered at the local hospital radio station, and enjoyed weekly yoga classes. I was sickeningly wholesome and unapologetically living life to the fullest.

But then everything went tits up. On Wednesday 8th February 2015, I woke up in the dead of night with overwhelming nausea. For someone who had only been physically sick twice in living memory (once after eating too many Crème Eggs at Brownies, and the other at university with food poisoning), this was unusual. I sat upright on the mattress, took a sip of water, and opened my window for a blast of cold air. *Not to worry,* my internal calming voice croaked. *It's probably dinner coming back on you. Maybe the cheese in my macaroni was off. Yeah, probably that.* I closed my eyes and tried to stop thinking of food.

Less than a minute later, I was hunched over my toilet bowl and vomiting blood. I recall looking at the maroon mess, so vividly contrasting against the white porcelain, and thinking: *OK, this isn't great.* I knew I needed to get this checked over and knew it probably couldn't wait until the morning. I didn't cry. I didn't panic. Instead, I did what any self-respecting millennial would do (?!) and took a photo on my iPhone in case a doctor needed to see it (chronic illness has provided me with dizzyingly high squeamish thresholds). Floating into autopilot, I flushed the last two minutes down the loo and started tidying the surrounding lino with some Dettol wipes.

Whilst pep-talking to my reflection in the bathroom mirror, I brushed my teeth to rinse out the worst of the metallic taste. I changed out of my jammies into a dress and tights, clipped on my wig and – don't try this at home, kids – *drove myself to A&E*. Why, you might ask, did I think getting in a car was anything like a good idea? I think the reason was two-fold: firstly, I didn't want the 'fuss' of an ambulance, and secondly, I genuinely thought driving would be the quickest way to get myself to the hospital. I should probably be retrospectively arrested.

With it being half three on a Wednesday morning in the Scottish Borders, A&E was deserted, so I was triaged immediately by a lovely nurse who guided me through to a side room and motioned for me to take a seat.

"And how much blood did you lose, do you think?" she asked, straightening out a pile of forms and circling some boxes.

"Ooooh, quite a lot," I replied, my speech becoming somewhat laboured as it required breath I now didn't seem to have.

"Mmm-hmm." She switched on a PC screen which illuminated the room, her neatly manicured fingers hovering above the keyboard. "But how much? A teaspoon? Tablespoon?"

"A mugful?" I offered, trying to think about how much blood I'd lost, before remembering my disturbingly diligent photography. I dug my phone out my pocket. "I've actually got a picture –"

Her hand flew up in haste. "Woah-ho-*no*. Just a description is fine."

"Imagine being sick, but instead of sick, it's, like, all blood."

Concern now glistened in her eyeballs. "We'll need to admit you, I think. Would you like a wheelchair to help you down the corridor?"

"Oh, no, it's ok. I'll be fine." I regretted my decision approximately ten seconds later as we started pacing down the corridor together to yet another room. Struggling to not faint under the bright lights – why can't they have mood lighting in hospitals? – I glanced at the time. Four in the morning, which was far too early to text Mum. When I eventually texted her at seven, both my parents immediately commenced the six-hour journey to see me. On reflection, receiving that text must have been their worst nightmare, and the drive down must have been agonisingly long.

An A&E consultant sent me to a ward upstairs for further investigation, and some kindly nurses found me a bed in a private suite. It was at this point, with the nondescript hospital issue gown on and an ID band taped round my wrist, that I grasped quite how far I'd drifted up shit creek without a paddle. Three hours later, a liver consultant confirmed that swollen veins (varices) had developed in my oesophagus (caused by portal vein hypertension, caused by liver cirrhosis, caused by AIH) and had bled. I was 'lucky' to have not suffered a more serious, or even fatal, haemorrhage.

Within the space of a few hours, my adrenaline rush had evaporated into the ether, leaving me feeling a woozy kind of unwell that I hadn't experienced before. It was an emptiness, or more specifically a weakness, where even breathing – that one basic life skill – felt like too much effort. My body had finally cottoned on that something wasn't right, but it didn't have the mental resources to work out what, exactly. Knowing I was somewhere safe, my body entered its low-battery, power-saving zone. At this point, all I could think about was what I needed to do, or take, to feel normal again. IV antibiotics? Shoot me up. Fluid drip? Straight into the jugular, please. Anaesthetic? Knock me out.

What I ended up needing to stop the bleeding was an endoscopy (as a reminder, this is a long thin flexible camera delicately shoved down the throat) but with an extra add-on procedure called 'banding'. Put simply, banding involves a fancy bit of kit being attached to the endoscope, which is then used to apply little rubber-band-type things over the swollen bits of vein. These rubber bands cause the varices to ulcerate and then heal over in a few days. Ultimately, the varices become smaller (or to use the posh term, 'eradicated'). This reduces, but not necessarily eliminates, the risk of bleeding.[38]

I was discharged a couple of days later, feeling like shite warmed up. The procedure itself made my chest feel like it had been used as a dancefloor for a line dancing class where everyone wore steel-capped boots. I recall sitting in the back seat of the car waiting for my parents to finish a Tesco shop and determining that I was in the most pain I had ever been in.

Inwardly breathing anything more than a shallow intake of air, or even swallowing saliva, was followed by an immense burning. Anaemic, with the rims of my eyes a translucently pale pink, I could hardly muster up the wherewithal for conversation. Over the course of the next day, I passed out when I got up from the sofa – one of two fixed resting points, along with my bed – to pee. Anything other than sleeping required energy reserves that were already well into the red overdraft. The thought of food made my stomach churn and my chest roar with pain. I was afraid to drink tea in case it burst ulcers that were trying to heal up (I don't think this is even possible, but nonetheless I still had visions of it happening).

Two days later, tests showed that my haemoglobin (a component of blood) levels were falling off a cliff. It was

---

[38] Science is so *fricking clever*, isn't it? Obviously, I'd rather all this wasn't going on inside my body, but still, it's mind-blowingly cool. Go science!

decided that I needed two blood transfusions.[39] Yet the party was far from over; later that night, I noticed that my stomach was increasingly bloated. What I tried to tell myself was just a wee bit of flab from not moving much was actually ascites (reminder for those who skipped the biology chapter: this is the formal name for the problem wherein fluid is not cleared by your liver and instead gets diverted to the easiest storage place, the abdomen, causing a tight and strained belly).

I was prescribed diuretics (medicines that make you pee like the Trevi fountain) and a low-salt diet to rid my belly of the fluid. Additionally, my liver inflammation markers started a meteoric rise, resulting in a return of the infamous high-dose steroids to get the numbers back under control. In the space of a few days, my liver had 180-ed from 'compensated' (working) to 'decompensated' (not working).

To all intents and purposes, my life seemed to be fast transforming into a shitshow. There came a point where there was so much uncertainty flying around, with things changing so quickly, and me feeling so out of control over what was going to happen, that I just shut down the part of me that even tried to worry. Anxiety would rear its ugly head inside my own – *maybe this is the time I'll need to be fast-tracked for transplant, because my liver can't swerve away again from its Icarus-esque brush with the danger zone* – but something in my brain decided to shut it down. It was as if my body was just refusing to give anxiety the headspace in amongst the other landmines going off.

Worries I had fretted over in the week before my bleed – the undercurrent of feeling a bit lost in my work, relationships and life plans – now seemed trivial and irrelevant. The very

[39] I am eternally grateful to the people whose blood donations quite honestly saved my life and, within hours, made me feel exponentially better. Please keep donating blood if you are able to.

foundations of my life priorities were shaken, and everything became so much simpler. I was buzzing just to still be alive.

Over the next few weeks, the steroids really kicked in. My inflammation markers came down, and my ascites cleared. My varices resolved and would remain monitored with annual endoscopy checkups. Life slowly returned to what it had been before, in many ways. Yet I felt that something fundamental in my own attitude had changed.

If someone had told teenaged me that I was going to wake up on my own in the middle of the night and spew up blood, I'd have crumpled into a corner and hyperventilated into a paper bag. What I find most interesting is that, when shit hit the fan, I didn't freeze in fear. I didn't have a total meltdown. I'm not trying to show off how serene I was, even in the face of something scary, or implying I would have been any less proud of myself if I had, for example, suffered a panic attack. There's no way of knowing if I'd react in the same way if this was to happen again. But it's worth noting that, sometimes, the things we *think* we are not capable of are actually well within the remit of our capabilities. We should give ourselves more credit, because often we are a lot stronger than we realise.

Indeed, even writing about it now, I struggle to wrap my head around the capacity of the body to dissociate and go into survival mode. The strength of the instinct to stay alive causes me to reflect on the mind state of those whose mental health conspires to override it. The desperation they face must be so unbelievably awful to swim against that magnetic force.

I've heard some women say that childbirth provided them with a belief in the primal, powerful capabilities of their own bodies. In a slightly similar way, it took a flirtatious dance with death for me to prove to myself that I am a tough cookie. I started, albeit tentatively, to have confidence in my abilities.

Would I have reached that stage with age alone? Possibly, but I think my oesophageal bleed fast-forwarded the process. Like a successful childbirth, I've mostly forgotten the trauma of my bleed and been blessed with the positive reminder that life is too short and too precious to waste. So, crank up another 90s tune – I'll plump for Republica's '*Ready to Go*' – and go live it.

# ON GRATITUDE

It's possibly a by-product of an adolescence spent watching one too many Final Destination films on Channel 4, but I spend a lot of time these days thinking of the ways, not necessarily health-related, in which a life could be forever changed.

When driving behind one of those articulated lorries piled high with logs, a warning from nowhere bleats in my inner ear: *"Keep your distance, Kirsty. You never know quite how secure those logs are in there."* I'm the doomsayer who studies aeroplane safety cards, dutifully taking my earphones off whilst air hostesses do the emergency exit macarena. Some might say I'm an obsessive overthinker on constant verge of an anxiety attack; I prefer the term *mindful of risk*.

My two close shaves with death (thus far) are as follows:

1. Driving Gladys, my Ford Fiesta, along the treacherous A7 on a particularly rainy day with a particularly heavy load of shopping distributed particularly unevenly in the boot.

Coming round a tight corner, Gladys aquaplaned onto the other side of the road. If there had been a car on the opposite carriageway, we would all have been on a one-way trip to the morgue. Did my life flash before my eyes? Not quite. I was too preoccupied trying to work out how to control my steering wheel, which began to freestyle spin like something out of Grand Theft Auto.
2. My aforementioned oesophageal bleed, where I was too focussed on cleaning up my bathroom lino to be recapping my major milestones.

As much as we might soothe ourselves with lullabies of self-determination and pretences of control, it is often just pure luck that keeps our lives the way we like them to be. Thinking about the intrinsic randomness, the powerlessness and the fragility of it all for too long, and you risk drowning in a bottomless pit of anxiety.

In my two close shaves, the contemplation of how narrowly my own demise had been avoided didn't fully kick in until sometime later. Ever since my internal bleed, I've maintained a baseline level of gratitude that hasn't dipped all that much. It's waxed and waned, for sure, but overall, I've noticed that each time I've been super unwell, this sense of gratitude perversely becomes a little bit stronger. I often wonder if it's a function of my personality – I'm quite stubborn, and the more challenging something is, the more determined I become to not let it get me down – but I think there's a more practical element to it, too.

During these times, I'm forced to really live in the moment. I take each hour as it comes, because feeling okay in the morning does not prevent my body taking a nosedive at noon. Every tiny scrap of progress – moving away from being *nil by mouth*, finishing the course of IV antibiotics, or getting my cannula removed – feels hard-won. In between being woken up for intermittent blood draws, I dream of nights free from beeping machines, settled in my own bed, with non-hospital issue loungewear and the blissful feel of unstarched bedsheets.

Nothing spurs on my ability to make plans for when I'll get better (because it's important to believe that I *will* get better) more than being hooked up to a fluids drip. As the clear liquid edges, centimetre by centimetre, into my veins, I think of all the things I want to do after escaping from the hospital prison: bracing strolls with my parents' dog on a far-flung Scottish beach, or curling up in my own armchair to delve into a good book with my eyesight not blurred from high-dose steroids.

A two-year long IBS[40] flare, which rendered me unable to confidently leave my house without an emergency Imodium, remains a highly effective memento to be grateful for every meal I can now eat without needing to rush to the toilet immediately after. I feel duty-bound, on behalf of all those people who can't get out the house or are lying ill in hospital, to make the most of life every single day. I know what it feels like to not be guaranteed a healthy tomorrow.

Thing is, nobody is guaranteed a tomorrow. Let this be a team reminder: go and do the things you want to do. Don't wait for next summer, or when you've got more money, or when you've lost weight, or gained a boyfriend. Have confidence in yourself, don't think about things too much. If you have good health, you're arguably one of the richest people on the planet.

Facing my mortality at an age when very few others were even considering the impact of their lifestyle on their *bank*

---

[40] Irritable bowel syndrome. Does what it says on the tin.

*balance*, let alone their longevity, was not something I was initially grateful for. Lecture-free afternoons spent poring over online articles about the prognosis of cirrhosis left me struggling to conjure up visions of a life beyond university.

Because, at 20, I only *notionally* understood the concept of aging. I had grown up with the privileged assumption that I would, of course, get older. It was bewildering to suddenly find myself swinging from this cosy viewpoint to one where that hazily-imagined future was scrubbed clean overnight, leaving a blank void which came with no instruction manual for how to colour it back in.

The truth is that every day, I'm still trying to find the right crayons, but I'm beginning to think that's the whole point. Being grateful doesn't mean I've reached a complete acceptance of my life situation, my health conditions and their impacts, and never complain or moan. I'm not donning orange robes, denying all material goods and heading out for 5am incantations at the local monastery with a trail of incense following in my wake. Sometimes, a shit situation is just shit. There's no upside, no positive spin.

But equally, I'm certainly not prepared to settle for less in any area of my life, whether that's my ambitions, dreams, relationships or healthcare. I still feel a drive to get what I want despite my illness, and I'd go so far as to say I'm motivated to do many of these things *as a direct result* of it.

It took a long time for that penny to drop, but now that it has, I even see myself as a little bit *more* deserving of good things. If something good happens, I try to enjoy it, and I take note of it. If something bad happens, I don't dwell on it, nor add it to what could quickly become a stacked-up pile of signs the universe is conspiring against me. Instead, I lower the threshold for treating myself kindly, as I would a friend.

And I don't mean to say I'm entitled to a paradise island off St Martinique purely because I've had to deal with health problems. Quite the opposite: it's the normality of the everyday, the monotonous backing vocals of life, that I try to take stock of. I'm talking about the perfect-temperature cup of tea in my favourite mug, or when that bus doesn't torpedo through the puddle at the side of the road next to me. Laughing so hard that I'm at risk of developing one-third of a six pack, or complimenting someone on their jumper and seeing their face light up. My favourite song playing on the radio on the way to work, making a baby chuckle, getting a nail polish stain out of white trousers, the stratospheric satisfaction of bleeding a radiator, or self-assembling anything from IKEA (especially when using a high heel as a makeshift hammer). Executing perfectly matched eyeliner. Breaking into freshly baked bread. Birdsong. A first date with – *imagine!* - good conversation.

The great thing about facing really shite situations is that a lot of the other annoying noise of life suddenly becomes only *slightly* shite, or even a wee bit comical. Rejected for a job after spending hours on the cover letter and three pounds on the bus fare to the interview? Ach well. They didn't deserve me anyways. That sucker punch in the guts upon realising I've somehow corrupted the Excel file at work? There'll be a backup somewhere on that infamous cloud. Stood up on a date outside a theatre in the pouring rain and instead drive to a McDonalds where I end up biting into a drive-thru McChicken burger instead of a McVeggie one, as per my order? Saved from an evening's tedious chat with an emotionally unavailable idiot.

Am I living my so-called best life? Probably not. But is

anyone, really? Is life best lived through serial highs, glossing over or avoiding any hint of problems or difficulties…or is it made more full, more worth living, with a wider spectrum of experiences? For me, enjoying life isn't about posting Instagram reels of cocktails in fancy restaurants overlooking city skylines as part of jet-set holidays to five-star boutiques, nor progressing up career ladders and making sure everyone knows about my latest promotion on the snoozefest that is LinkedIn. It's about taking the good stuff with the bad stuff and mixing it up as part of the amazingness of life – even if it doesn't all feel like the 'best time ever' when I'm going through it.

Whilst I may be pissed off at how liver disease and lupus and everything else continues to force readjustment of my life plans – what I wanted to do, who I wanted to be, and where I wanted to go – the way I live my life today is by virtue of that opportunity to readjust my perspective. Just as a life can change for the worse with a spin of the die, each new day brings with it potential for improvement, for advancement, for *good* change. The most powerful miracles, after all, are sometimes the ones happening every day without us even noticing, until we make a conscious effort to do so.

If a genie offered to swap my current life for a normal liver and a Genghis Khan-level army of white blood cells[41], would I say yes? Would I trade in the lessons I've learned and the viewpoints I now have? I am who I am because of my conditions, and I'm endlessly grateful for that. Therefore the answer, genie, is thanks, but I'll pass.

---

[41] White blood cells are a key component of a healthy immune system. My levels are very low.

# ON RESILIENCE AND VULNERABILITY

Pop music gets a bad rep. It's too mainstream, too cheesy. But even the cool dudes on BBC6Music cannot deny the indisputable fact that pop songs have a therapeutic magic all of their own. I'm sorry, but if you've not played Beyoncé on repeat for a solid three weeks post-break up, you really haven't lived. There's a reason why pop songs are, well, popular, and that reason is their lyrics can be applied to many life situations. For those two minutes of major chord inversions, the listener feels like they're *understood.*

What have Kelly Clarkson's *'What Doesn't Kill You (Makes You Stronger)'*, *'I Will Survive'* by Gloria Gaynor, Natasha Beddingfield's *'Unwritten'*, and Taylor Swift's *'Shake It Off'* got in common? A relentlessly catchy hook? Yes, but also an overarching theme of resilience, which is why these all feature on my 'Living With Autoimmune Disease' playlist.

Serious illness comes with its very own hard-won skillset. Ripping away the comfort blanket of a clean bill of health requires a PhD in adaptability, which was quite the ask when I had only just passed my Advanced Highers. Firstly, I had to quickly understand that I was, in fact, ill.

I had to adapt to taking new medicines that made my appearance change. Then there was the adapting to having new, sometimes quite serious, symptoms appearing, and learning to deal with them rationally. And *then* there was the requirement to adapt my decision-making processes, making good (but not necessarily easy) choices every single day: leaving parties early to get enough sleep whilst everyone else waxed lyrical about the legendary nights out for weeks afterwards, exercising when my sinews felt fit to melt with fatigue, fitting in appointments around lectures (and then, years later, work meetings), eating well when I really couldn't be bothered to cook after a long day. Maintaining good health habits demanded a crash-course in maturity.[42]

Despite adapting as well as could be expected, I soon learned that being a star patient doesn't prevent my health from nosediving. I'm now so used to being told bad news from doctors that I often don't quite believe it when things are normal. It feels *wrong.* Bad news is never easy to listen to, or to accept. But I do notice that I have an ability to process it more quickly and efficiently than I did when I was first diagnosed. I have learned, just about, how to recentre my thoughts – however stressed or angry or upset I might be – around the realisation that, in the grand scheme of the universe, any situation I face or emotion I feel is likely to be fleeting. The world continues to spin. There's usually a bigger picture to be seen.

The great thing is that this resilience often translates into

---

[42] Don't get me wrong, Little Miss Conformity here probably would have been health-conscious anyways, but the harsh truth is that if I wasn't, I likely would not be here.

other areas of my life. It's a cliché, but I really don't sweat the small stuff as much anymore. Compared to some of the showstoppers I've faced and lived through, I don't get too down about failures or disappointments. I'll give it my best shot, dust myself off, and try again.

Over the years, I've become *au fait* with metaphorical doors slamming in my face because of my health. A gap year travelling round far-flung exotic locations? Not unless I have a spare three grand for travel insurance. Long-haul flights? Quite risky when you might have an internal bleed with the change in pressure. Biological motherhood? Nope, nope, nope.

Yet for every door that closes, there have usually been two more that spring open in its place. Having liver disease has pinballed me into meeting a range of different people with whom I would otherwise never have had the privilege of engaging. I have been fortunate enough to meet countless diligent and fiercely intelligent charity workers, doctors, nurses and other healthcare staff, all valiantly trying to improve people's quality of life.

And then, of course, there's my fellow brothers and sisters in (tourniquet-ed) arms across all ages, races, illnesses, and social demographics. Illness – or indeed, more generally, human suffering – transcends borders, languages, religions, and cultures. This has been humbling; I've learnt that none of us, no matter how rich or how clever or how kind, are immune from life's difficulties. It's how people respond in the face of their difficulties, their resilience, that is the most inspiring bit.

Many people – people like you and me, working normal jobs, paying bills, cooking dinner, bleaching the toilet – choose day upon day to make positive out of what are undeniably shitty situations. They just get on with life as best they can and, in some special cases, endeavour to use their experience to make life better for someone else. There is something about illness which can bring out the best qualities in some humans. *These* are the people society should be celebrating, rather than the latest influencer who blatantly spews out paid adverts for the highest bidder.

Vulnerability, meanwhile, is a strange concept. Superficially, at least, a vulnerability makes us weak. Illness has made me feel vulnerable both physically, in terms of being sometimes unable to do what I would expect to be able to do as a young person, and also emotionally, in feeling like I have very little power or control over what is going on within my own body.

But *allowing* myself to be openly vulnerable – accepting that weakness and having the confidence to be open about it – has inadvertently brought about a strong sense of oneself. Only now do I understand that not any one of us is *without* some degree of vulnerability. Everyone is flawed, and it is these imperfections that act as the lowest common denominator to connect us.

Take, for example, the time when I was in an endoscopy waiting room with two older women. Having broken the awkward silence with a comment about the Saharan-level heat blasting out of what should have been an air-cooling unit[43], I learned that they were both in for their first ever sigmoidoscopies[44], and reassured them that the procedure was, in my experience, not too bad if they took all the sedation on offer. Their shoulders visibly de-hunched. The tension in the room dissipated. We eventually wound up chatting about the

[43] God loves the NHS for trying.

[44] A scope of the sigmoid colon and the lower bit of your large intestine.

problems post-menopausal women face in society and I learned things about cervical prolapse that even seasoned gynaecologists probably wouldn't be quite prepared for at half past three on a Thursday afternoon.

I digress. The point is that being vulnerable, being honest, and confronting fears head on can sometimes be refreshingly helpful. Having a chat whilst sitting down in paper pants, wrapped only in hospital-issue gowns is, it turns out, a great social leveller.

Being vulnerable allows pathways to open up to meet others with a shared lived experience. Regardless of the difference in symptoms or energy levels, this can bring about a sense of community which is often very hard to find. Nothing quite chimes like bonding over a shared hatred for prednisolone with someone who lives on a different continent.

Acknowledging its vulnerability has made me realise that my body is amazingly powerful. Despite a platelet level low enough to challenge a Hawaiian limbo dancer, it works well enough to let me live my life. There is not one day that goes by where I am not secretly in awe at how it puts up with it all.

# ON MY LIVER HEROES

As a fully paid-up (and possibly only) member of the *Love Your Liver* club, it feels only right for me to provide a whistlestop tour round a selection of the most interesting characters in the liver disease community over the last century.

It's a hard job to whittle down the list; I had to leave out cool dudes like Antoine Portal, who first noted the bleeding that occurs due to the presence of oesophageal varices in cirrhotic patients way back in 1770, and Francis Moore, who pioneered the first liver transplant (in a dog) in 1958.[xlv] I've neglected to include Roger Williams and Sir Roy Calne, the super-intelligent duo who kicked off *human* liver transplantation in the UK. (What's more, Williams published over 2,750 papers on liver disease and trained over 600 doctors and scientists on liver care[xlvi], whilst Calne identified the first immunosuppressive drug to prevent organ rejection post-transplant.[xlvii])

There are so many *ordinary* liver heroes, too, who don't necessarily have prestigious awards or breakthrough discoveries but are nonetheless helping in their own way to advancing our understanding of liver disease. From patients who are trialling new treatments or raising awareness of liver health, to the doctors, researchers and scientists who strive for excellence within hepatology, there are great people doing even greater work who will probably never get the appreciation they deserve. Then there are all the families, friends and supporters who help to make the liver community a generally welcoming place. So whilst not all heroes wear capes, all *my* heroes understand the importance of a healthy liver.

### *Dame Sheila Sherlock (1918-2001)*[xlviii]

With one of the best alliterative names going, this Dubliner was a trailblazer in the world of hepatology, and moreover medicine more generally, in the 1950s. Born in 1918, Sherlock was raised in a single-parent household and received a grant to allow her to continue her academic studies beyond secondary school. Her applications to study medicine were rejected from every English university, but Sherlock was accepted into the University of Edinburgh.[45] It was here she eventually graduated top of her class, winning the sought-after Ettles Scholarship, in 1941.

Despite evident academic excellence, she found herself unable to start an internship at the Edinburgh's Royal Infirmary. Why, then, was the top student unable to partake in what would surely be an obvious progression and good use of her skills and intelligence? Was she a communist spy? Was she found to have cheated in her finals? Did she set fire to the

---

[45] I'm biased, what with it being my *alma mater*, but the UoE admissions board clearly knows excellent potential when it sees it. Though, like many other medical schools of the era, Edinburgh required that female medical students were to undertake dissections in a separate room from the males.

medical school on her last day? Of course not. Naturally, Sheila Sherlock couldn't start an internship at the hospital because *she was a woman*, and the infirmary didn't have any live-in quarters for females.[xlix]

Undeterred, Sherlock took up a locum position with a general practitioner in Perth before she realised that she craved a more academic role with clinical research. This would involve work in an academical institution, and these jobs were not generally on offer to women. Recognising Sherlock's brilliance, James Learmouth, the then-Professor of Surgery at the University of Edinburgh (and the clinician who performed surgery on King George VI), offered her the role of Assistant Lecturer in Surgery. This allowed her to assist at operations and fulfil the role of House Surgeon in all but name.

Yet this placement confirmed to Sherlock that surgery was not where her future lay, and instead she set her sights on research. Under the advice of Learmouth, she moved to London to work as a house physician at Hammersmith Hospital under another eminent medic, Professor John McMichael. McMichael, a Scotsman whose *alma mater* was also University of Edinburgh, employed Sherlock in the then-newly opened Postgraduate Centre.[l] (McMichael was one of the first doctors to start using liver biopsies during the early years of World War Two, and he shared his technique with Sherlock.)

The limited scope of global liver knowledge at this point in her career cannot be underestimated; the concept of hepatology as a standalone speciality was very much in its infancy. Liver function tests weren't yet routine practice, biopsies weren't a core part of the liver problem toolbox, and little was known about cirrhosis other than it was usually linked with excessive alcohol intake.

In 1943, a groundbreaking joint publication on the pathology of acute hepatitis between Sherlock, McMichael and another doctor called Henry Dible helped to pave the way for a funded study of the biochemistry of liver disorders and, in the immediate post-war years, an examination of the effects of malnutrition (which was still widespread in Germany at that time) on liver health. Sherlock, meanwhile, soon became a leading expert on liver biopsies. By the age of 30, she had successfully navigated her way to being Honorary Consultant Physician at Hammersmith. She was a wee bit like the Taylor Swift of hepatology in the 1950s, but without all the due recognition.

Sherlock was later given her own liver unit at the Royal Free Hospital in London. The unit went on to generate a formidable research output, contributing extensively to the field of liver health. Amongst her achievements was her introduction of needle liver biopsies, which allowed patients who were too ill for general anaesthesia to undergo a less-invasive biopsy process.

The unit soon attracted leading hepatologists globally, and advancements in the fields of drug-induced liver damage, portal hypertension, ascites, viral hepatitis, liver transplantation, the use of endoscopic methods for treating varices, autoimmune liver disease (and, importantly, the use of steroids in its treatment) and bilirubin metabolism were made. In 1966, Sherlock contributed towards creating a diagnostic test for what is now understood to be primary biliary cholangitis.[li]

She was the Royal College of Physicians' first female vice president, and her first textbook on liver conditions – *Diseases of the Liver and Biliary System* – was published in 1954 and thereafter translated into six languages. It's somewhat unsurprising that she was listed as one of the world's top ten most cited female scientists of the 1980s by *Scientist* magazine.

On a personal level, Sherlock was something of a formidable force of nature – a "tornado", as one of her contemporaries described her. She was known to have the ability to send colleagues to the depths of despair with her literal tearing up of research paper drafts. Some of her clinical practices were, euphemistically, *of their time*, and would not pass the stringent ethics tests of today. Patient consent to testing was rarely offered, for example. Dr Maurice Papworth took aim at her methods in his 1969 book about clinical research trials, pithily named 'Human Guinea Pigs'.

Yet this should not cast a shadow over the incredible work that Sherlock facilitated and carried out; without her tenacious approach to research, the hepatology landscape would look very different today.

### *Dr Juan Rodés (1938- 2017)*[lii]

Juan Rodés was the head of hepatology services at the Hospital Clinic of Barcelona. At the start of his career, after completing his medical degree at the Medical School of Barcelona, he received a government grant to travel to Paris and began working with Professor Jacques Caroli (an eminent hepatologist) at the esteemed Saint Antoine hospital. It was here that Rodés began to see the potential for clinical research – and specifically *liver* research – within a hospital structure.

With this experience under his belt, Rodés returned to Spain to establish his own Liver Unit in Barcelona. Shortly after, he helped to setup the first ICU in Spain dedicated to treating liver disease patients. The theory behind this, according to

Rodés, was that the liver patients were best served by doctors who were specifically trained to the nuances of liver disease and its complications, and who were interested in the mechanisms of the disease and keen to understand and optimise the treatments to benefit patients the most. It seems obvious now, but only a few decades ago, the concept of patient-focussed care was still very much in its infancy, and Rodés' focus on the importance of collaboration was certainly innovative.

Rodés' output from the Barcelona Liver Unit significantly advanced the treatment of various complications of cirrhosis. He also conducted ground-breaking research into hepatocellular carcinoma; algorithms that were developed at the unit to assist in treating liver cancer are still used worldwide.

In 2015, as an advisor to the Spanish Ministry of Health, Rodés spearheaded negotiations to provide patients with affordable access to newly available hepatitis C antiviral drugs. He was given a limited timeframe in which to devise a plan of action, which necessitated complex global supply chain discussions with pharmaceutical companies and political leaders.[liii]

Throughout his career, and specifically during his tenure at the Barcelona Liver Unit, Rodés emphasised the importance of teamwork, both with his research colleagues in Spain and with other hepatologists worldwide. He never sought recognition for being the person to initiate the Unit's establishment, preferring to claim it was collaborative effort. He was a grade-A team player whose hard work, sense of humility and minimal-fuss approach made a significant impact on the global liver disease community.

### *Gertrude Elion (1918 – 1999)*[liv]

Full disclaimer: I'm chief cheerleader for this lady because:

1. She studied chemistry. (I, too, studied chemistry.)
2. She worked in Research & Development (R&D) for Smith Kline Beecham, a company which later became GSK. (I worked for GSK. It is my opinion that they are a great company, with smart people trying to improve life for those with rare diseases including lupus and liver disease.)
3. She helped contribute towards the synthesis of two of the drugs which have been used to prolong and improve the quality of my life. (And…this is where our similarities end.)

Like Sheila Sherlock, Elion was born in 1918. She grew up in New York with her parents, who were Eastern European migrants, and her grandfather joined them from Russia when she was three. Elion was close to him as she grew up, and witnessing his protracted and painful death from stomach cancer when she was 15 had a profound impact on her, ultimately becoming the motivation for her life's work.

The 1929 financial crash left her family penniless, and despite Elion graduating with a chemistry degree from Hunter College (a school offering free tuition for the academically gifted), she was unable to afford to attend graduate school immediately afterwards. Fellowships were not on offer to women at the time, because…*oh, wait.* There was no valid reason.

Undeterred and armed with her degree in chemistry, Elion set out to find work. And find work she did, but not in a laboratory. After a short stint as a secretary, she later found a temporary job as a biochemistry teacher and then after that, took on an unpaid role as a laboratory assistant which led to a paid position.

Saving up her wages, she manged to enrol in graduate classes at New York University, where she graduated with a master's degree in 1941, notably the only woman in her chemistry class. As World War Two steadily depleted the global stock of male chemists[46], Elion was afforded an opportunity to join the ranks of scientists, firstly as a food chemist and then later in research at Johnson & Johnson.

Finding herself wanting more from her work, in 1944 she found a job assisting the eminent George Hitchings at a pharmaceutical company called Burroughs Welcome, where they would collaborate on a new, forward-thinking approach to drug development. Rather than use trial-and-error, as was routine practice at the time, Elion and Hitchings preferred to use a more rational, evidence-based approach. The duo successfully synthesised two compounds that could interfere with the lifecycle of a malicious type of cell found in leukaemia patients. However these drugs were highly toxic, often causing more harm than good to the patient. This frustrated and upset Elion in equal amounts. A near-relative of these drugs, called 6-mercaptopurine (or 6-MP) was discovered not too long after by Elion. This, when combined with other drugs, was found to more effectively treat childhood leukaemia.

Elion continued to make further discoveries, including azathioprine, which is one of the medicines I took for many years as a cornerstone immunosuppressant in my drug regime. Azathioprine suppresses immune response and was one of the

---

[46] The war also brought about the death of Elion's partner at the time, from an infectious disease for which there was no antibiotics available to treat. It is said that Elion never recovered from his loss and never married.

first drugs which facilitated organ transplantation back in the early 1960s.

Not content with her steaming progress, Elion was determined to enhance the properties of her earlier discovery (6-MP). Her tenacity paid off; in 1963, allopurinol was developed. This drug, a derivative of 6-MP, was found to reduce the body's production of uric acid, a key factor in the causes of gout (a condition that can prove fatal for cancer patients).[lv]

This achievement alone would be enough to satisfy the career ambitions of any drug discovery scientist, but Elion's successes were far from ending. In 1977, she developed an antiviral drug called acyclovir, the first drug ever developed to specifically fight a virus. Prior to this, many doctors disbelieved that viruses could ever be targeted, as they thought that any drug with the ability to do this would be too toxic for the body to metabolise safely. Elion proved them wrong, for acyclovir was – and still is – a wonder-drug used to treat cases of shingles and herpes simplex. This heralded a new goldrush of antiviral therapy development, which later opened the floodgates for treatments for AIDS (which, in a nice roundabout fashion, is a key therapeutic focus of GSK today).

Elion's name is printed on the patent for a staggering 45 different life-enhancing drugs. The painstaking work that goes into developing a new drug, checking the right dose, making sure it's not toxic and does no greater harm than good, cannot be overstated. To have done this time and time again is nothing short of genius. Yet despite mastering the art of drug formulation, Elion never forgot the driving force behind her work. Poignantly, she would store prized letters which were sent to her from grateful patients. Upon receiving the Nobel Prize in 1988, she said that:

*"What we were aiming at was getting people well, and the satisfaction of that is much greater than any prize you can get."*

People nowadays are perhaps a little too quick to paint 'big pharma' corporations as monstrous beasts borne of a special breed of capitalism that feeds off the misfortune and ill health of others. I believe that the reality is more nuanced. Yes, there is money to be made from healthcare, because we all need healthcare, and any service that is necessary (and necessarily done safely) comes at a price.

If we want to attract the best people and brightest minds to work towards facilitating medical discoveries, then we need to pay them well. But at the heart of pharmaceuticals – and I do genuinely believe this – there lies not exclusively an EBITDA financial target to meet at year end, or stakeholder returns to inflate a CEO's pension pot. There, too, lies a group of fiercely intelligent people like Elion, who want to make other people's lives better. People who genuinely want to improve the world we live in.

Elion received the 'Nobel Prize for Physiology or Medicine' in 1988 along with Hitchings and another researcher, James Black, for the development of their new rational approach to R&D. They changed the way drugs were synthesised and consequently paved the way for decades of enhancements and innovation thereafter. Whilst she died aged 81 in 1999, Elion's work lives on in the patients who take her drugs in their millions, every single day. She has saved countless lives and will continue to do so for generations in the future. Thank you, Gertrude!

## *Thomas Starzl (1926-2017)*[lvi]

Like Elion, the plight of a close family member (his mother) due to cancer determined the career path of a young Thomas Starzl, who went on to become known as the "father of modern transplantation".

Born in Iowa, Starzl later went on to perform the first ever liver transplant in Denver on the 1 March 1963. The recipient, three-year-old Bennie Solis, was a child who suffered from biliary atresia. Starzl and his team at the University of Colorado had prepared for the human liver transplant by performing over two hundred liver transplants in dogs[47] prior to the operation. Unfortunately, Bennie died from haemorrhage. Dissection proved to be very difficult due to high-pressure venous systems caused by portal hypertension.

Being 1963, there were few pharmaceutical options available to lessen the catastrophic blood loss, and Bennie's death led to a flurry of research into how to deal with clotting problems in severe liver disease.[lvii] Starzl's team recruited an expert physician, Kurt von Kaulla, who ultimately helped to develop a variety of agents to clot the blood in future liver transplantation procedures.[lviii]

Starzl went on to perform five further unsuccessful transplants until a voluntary cease in operations was agreed for the next three and a half years. In 1967, Starzl performed the first transplant with long-term survival – a nineteen-year-old girl called Julie Rodriguez who had a transplant as treatment for a hepatoblastoma. Julie survived for a further 400 days but ultimately passed away from a recurrence of the primary

[47] The dogs used in these experimental surgeries were euthanised afterwards. Starzl later noted that, *"It really bothers me in many respects to realise what a tremendous price was paid by dogs to allow transplantation...I couldn't do that again."*

tumour in her liver.[lix]

Starzl later transferred to working in the University of Pittsburgh, which went on to become one of the most prolific transplant centres globally. He developed therapeutic regimens whereby azathioprine and prednisone were used together to improve the success of liver transplantation. In 1966, the transplant institute there was named after Starzl himself. He went on to be the first liver transplant surgeon to use an immunosuppressant called cyclosporin in the 1970s[lx], and was a key advocate for the use of another immunosuppressant, tacrolimus, in transplant clinical practice from the 1990s[lxi] – advances which arguably revolutionised the world of organ transplantation.

Starzl contributed to over 3000 publications, and his ground-breaking work both in immunosuppressive therapies and organ preservation has profound and far-reaching impact on liver disease patients today.

### *Elena Baltacha (1983 – 2014)*[lxii]

Elena Baltacha (known as 'Bally') was a professional tennis player who lived with primary sclerosing cholangitis (PSC). Whilst Baltacha was born in Ukraine, she moved to Scotland aged six, growing up in Perth and latterly in Paisley, where her dad was a professional football player.

Aged 19, after a year of unexplained illness which kept her away from several high-profile tennis competitions, Baltacha was told that she had a form of liver disease. She was subjected to two liver biopsies in order to confirm the exact cause of her problems. One specialist suggested that she harboured a secret alcohol addiction and was "drinking more than George Best".

She said of her PSC diagnosis, which came at the same time as her rise through the ranks of the UK tennis circuit:

*"I cried solidly for days. I'd been playing well, people were telling me how talented I was, and I thought it was my time."*[lxiii]

On doctor's orders to rest for half a year, her future as a professional tennis player was looking increasingly uncertain. Undeterred, she focussed on building a healthy lifestyle and was soon back on the courts in 2004. As someone who can't keep a tennis ball on the court, I have the greatest admiration not only for Baltacha's sporting prowess, but also the sheer determination she had to achieve her goals. Of her liver condition, she said:

*"…[it's] still there, but I push it to the back of my mind…I've never used my health as an excuse. In a way, it's helped to give me another level of mental toughness."*

She later became the highest-ranked female singles player to come out of Scotland, smashing her way to British Number 1, a position she held on and off throughout 2002-2012. Her career-high position was World Number 49; she won 11 International Tennis Federation singles titles and went on to become a patron for the Children's Liver Disease Foundation – all whilst managing a chronic health condition.

When an Icelandic volcanic ash cloud grounded European flights in 2010, Baltacha found herself stranded at a competition in South Africa with a dwindling drug supply. Did she do a McEnroe and smash her racket off the clay courts in frustration at her health condition getting in the way of her living her life? No, she did not. She calmly rearranged a restock of the meds at her next tennis competition in Rome. I think this is proof, if more was needed, of the resilience this lady had.

Tragically, she was diagnosed with liver cancer just a few weeks after she retired from professional tennis. This cancer led to her premature death, aged 30, in 2014. Elena was nothing short of inspirational, and I continue to use her example of living life to the fullest as a blueprint for overcoming my own challenges. She said it best herself:

*"I want to show that liver disease doesn't have to end your dreams. Through hard work and burning desire you can still be successful."*

# ON MEDICS

Once a quarter, my psyche enters what could be referred to as an 'MLC' (mini-life-crisis). MLCs are triggered by events ranging from being ghosted on Tinder through to being told I will need to return to hospital for a repeat banding endoscopy in eight weeks' time. MLCs last anywhere between two hours and five days, during which time the versions of my personality[48] conspire together to forensically and painstakingly ruminate over every single life choice made up to that point.

Should I have left school after my Standard Grades and taken up a trade? (*No* – Risk-Assessor Kirsty butts in quickly – *because you would not be physically able to lift baths as a plumber, and you would likely electrocute yourself as an electrician.*) Why didn't I move to London straight after graduation? (Financial Advisor Kirsty steps to the fore - *because as a Scot it would be against your national religion to pay more than a grand per month for the privilege of a shared flat in Zone 4 furnished with black mould.*)

---

[48] Don't worry. I don't *think* I've got a personality disorder.

One of the more daring suggestions pitched in, time and time again, during these mental crucifixions from the sidelines of my mind is that all my career doubts would have been quashed if I'd chosen medicine as a vocation. (*You should have been a doctor*, Career Coach Kirsty chastises my 17-year-old, UCAS-application-making self. *You had the grades. You had the focus. You had the empathy. You'd be more fulfilled now if you'd done medicine.)* Thankfully, during these moments, Reality Checker Kirsty baseball-bats this idea right straight out of the field.

There is, of course, a list longer than the Dead Sea Scrolls of reasons why I couldn't have been a doctor:

1. I'm immunosuppressed. Ergo, working in a hospital, or any other healthcare setting near ill people, is not particularly conducive to my staying well.
2. Because of (1), I'm only full-of-the-milk-of-human-kindness if the human I'm being kind to is full of vaccines and free from viral illness. If people so much as blow their nose without using anti-bac afterwards, I ensure to avoid any surfaces they touch. If someone was to cough directly in my face, I could not be held responsible for my retaliating actions.
3. I didn't study biology in school. What's more, I'm not convinced I'm academically bright enough to have coped with the demands of medical school. I earned good grades through hard work, not natural aptitude.
4. I hate confrontation. Nine times out of ten, I'll wind up with heart palpitations if someone so much as raises their voice on public transport.
5. The workload would probably kill me. If I don't sleep well, I am knocked out for the next few days. Mixed in with shift working, the exhaustion would likely spell disaster for my mental and physical health.
6. I can't stand people who moan without good reason,

but doctors can't tell their hypochondriac patients to get lost, can they?

The bottom line is that the world is a better place for me not being a medic, in the same way as everyone is safer now that I'm not doing experiments in a chemical laboratory.[49] But spending so much time in hospital settings has made me reflect on my experiences with those who *do* chose medicine as a career (or more accurately, it would seem, as a lifestyle choice).

Doctors and nurses have borne witness to the most intimate parts of me, both physically and, increasingly as the years go on, emotionally. I've sat beside my liver consultant as we pore over a screen displaying pictures of "juicy" veins in my oesophagus, I've been handed a pack of Kleenex by a gynaecologist after breaking down with worry about getting my IUD inserted due to insertion horror stories on Reddit (mine was absolutely fine, if anyone else is worried), and I've seen the unmistakable horror in a junior doctor's eyes after they accidentally pierced through the back of my vein during a blood test, leaking a literal Red Sea onto the white lino floor.

Chronic illness laughs in the face of discretion, and there isn't much room for holding back when it comes to my consultants. They review the results of my sub-gastrointestinal biopsies, they provide reassurance that the irritating under-boob rash is just a fungal infection, they know the results of my latest HPV smear, they know my relationship status, and issue the prescriptions which keep me alive.

It's strange to know that a small collection of people who I have never spoken to outside of an NHS setting know my

[49] One time I accidentally pin-pricked myself with the needle of a pipe that was being used to bubble nitrogen gas through a solution. Nitrogen gas is deployed in the U.S. to execute death row inmates. I am the world's worst chemist.

bowel habits, blood type, BMI and birthday. It's clinically transactional, but bizarre, nonetheless. The only way I accept this duality is knowing that I'm not their only patient, and they're legally bound to not tell anyone else my inside leg measurement.

Like good friends, it's important to appreciate good doctors when you are lucky enough to have them. Like any other occupation, there are healthcare practitioners who are excellent at their jobs, and there are some who just simply weren't cut out for the path they've chosen to embark on, but have stuck to it regardless.

Everyone has a story to tell about a medic who was patronising, or dismissive, or just down-right rude. Those stories resonate, for sure; I've had my fair share. Nothing has made me feel more like a total freak of nature than the time I phoned the GP for thrush medication whilst being on a two-week course of antibiotics, only to be told by the nurse, "oh, so *you're* the girl with the rare Strep infection. Yes, we were discussing that when the swab result came back in. We were all quite shocked. Never seen that before." At the end of the call, I hung up, cried to my Mum for a bit, and then joined a Teams meeting at work like nothing had happened.

But it's important to remember that doctors and nurses are failingly human (even if a small minority of them might think they are of God-like rank). They still have personalities, despite years of training to beat out prejudices and gloss over with a sheen of professionalism. They are just as prone to mistakes, forgetting things, getting upset or frustrated or despondent as the rest of us mere mortals.

The key difference is that, for most occupations, the output isn't life or death. Those of us who aren't clinically trained can have a bad day safe in the knowledge that our worst outcome is likely to be a client negotiation divebombing into failure. For doctors, the burden of responsibility is far greater.

And therein lies the rub: society likes to think that doctors are the miracle workers of the modern age and, similar to the unrealistic expectations heaped on modern medicine, can provide an answer to every problem. When we go to the doctor, we expect them to know what's gone wrong and prescribe something to fix it (or at least confirm what we've self-diagnosed using a combination of Google and a lack of six years in medical school).

The danger with this portrayal is that it sets an unreachable expectation of our healthcare system. Whilst they can be incredibly knowledgeable and have unrivalled, invaluable experience in treating lots of patients with similar conditions, doctors are not machines. They don't know it all, and as far as I'm aware, they've never claimed to, either. We've just grown to expect it.

There have been times when a doctor cannot provide a straight-forward 'yes' or 'no' to my question without three asterisks for disclaimers or caveats. Sometimes no specialist from any department can explain definitively why my body has reacted in a certain way; instead, a few specialists will each offer some guesswork and leave me to decide who best to believe. Slipping into the gaps of specialist knowledge is a really uncomfortable place to be.

It's a bit like childhood in some ways; you grow up cocooned by the unwavering belief that everyone older than you must know what they're doing. Then it dawns on you as you grow older, when it's *your* generation carrying the weight of the world, that nobody really has a bloody clue what they're doing. They're just doing their best with the knowledge they have.

The best doctors are the ones who admit their knowledge gaps and limitations, but nonetheless guide you to face the uncertainty as a team. These doctors support you with the sense that they'll be on hand to work through the problems together.

As much as people love to complain about not being able to get a GP appointment, I can assure you that leapfrogging in priority at your local surgery is not a warm, cosy feeling. After my lupus diagnosis, I went from being an unexceptional patient with only a history of childhood asthma to being blacklisted and in need of a same-day callback if I ever phoned reception. Having a concoction of serious conditions and being immunocompromised means that some GPs won't touch me with an insulated barge pole in case they prescribe the wrong thing or miss something critically important in their evaluation. Whilst this is objectively scary and frustrating, it's understandable and ultimately reassuring. They, too, are accepting the limits of their expertise.

Consultants, on the other hand, are *au fait* with the intricacies of their specialist condition and therefore naturally confident in making more complex decisions. This difference in approach led to a situation not long after my liver disease diagnosis whereby a GP phoned me in a blind panic after my blood results come back with a platelet level of 30 (normal range is around 150-450). The GP then called the consultant haematologist, who informed them politely that he wouldn't really flinch unless the reading got down to single figures. It would, however, have been more helpful if the GP had done this *prior* to phoning me, because in the interim, I was on the edge of a nervous breakdown wondering if my veins were going to spontaneously collapse.

Whilst the blasé attitude of some consultants holds the potential to be reassuring, the reality is a little more nuanced. The danger is that these specialist doctors can become so accustomed to the big, dangerous, life-threatening stuff that it sometimes feels like they forget that the day-to-day reality of living with serious conditions, even when things are stable, can be very bloody frightening.

To some extent, as much as consultants live and breathe the conditions, even the best ones won't ever be able to fully '*get it*'. It's unreasonable to expect them to, because only when one is in the throes of living with the disease can the far-reaching effects be understood. It's probably even harder to understand because some patients (me included) put on brave faces in the consulting rooms and potentially give the impression that it's much easier to live a life with the condition than the reality may be.

It's not just the more obvious encroachments on life such as pain, which most people have some experience of and can therefore relate to. It's in the thousand other life-sucking mechanisms with which illness operates. It's in the needing an endless toolbox of coping strategies, such as strategising for how best to tell my boss that I might be put forward for transplant assessment soon. It's in the being denied critical illness insurance for a mortgage (in case I'm unable to work in future[50]) because I'm considered statistically likely to drop dead at any moment, or the mental gymnastics of establishing whether a wave of nausea is a viral bug that will pass in a few weeks, or the early warning signs of another oesophageal bleed.

---

[50] I am very privileged to be able to buy a flat, too.

The ways that health conditions creep like a poison ivy into the crevasses of daily life simply can't be explained in textbooks, yet it's these everyday problems, the challenges which no prescription can ease, that are often the most impactful.

I believe that it would be very difficult, impossible even, for a doctor to have the emotional reserve to fully grasp all this whilst being able to do their job well. Similarly, patients won't ever fully be able to understand what goes on behind the scenes from a doctor's perspective, and it's probably just as well. If I knew about all the things that could go wrong, I would probably melt with anxiety.

The bottom line is that medics don't have the time to deal with the stuff that isn't going to kill me directly. The NHS can't provide me with specialist travel insurance, and there's no Crystal Ball department for evidence that I'll still be able to work in a year or two. Patient support groups and charities help address some of the practical life problems, but there still exists a very isolating gap between the realm of the patient and that of the medic.

What, then, makes the ideal doctor? Does such a thing exist? I think they do, because I've met some, and I've got them on my team. Doctors are paid to be professional and remain somewhat detached, but in my mind, being a good doctor entails a dollop of genuine care about each of your patients. Good doctors should empathise, but not patronise. They listen, but hold firm in their rationality. The best doctors are honest, but not unfeeling. They talk with their patients from a position of equality, wherein one half of the partnership has the advantage of expert clinical knowledge, and the other has the advantage of lived experience.

Patients are not just statistics. Whilst clinical data drives treatment choices, I think it's important for doctors to recognise that being told you're *statistically likely* to be okay is as reassuring as hearing Captain Smith of the Titanic say that the *"ship could be cut crosswise in three places, and each piece would float"*.[lxiv]

Talking of ships, I prefer my doctors to be more like co-captains of the metaphysical boat of my body. They are experts whose opinions I trust and who I can bounce my questions and thoughts off. Whilst patient input on treatment options is all well and good, sometimes having the ultimate decision on the 'next step' in your plan can be overwhelming. Putting five medics in a room to discuss a case will result in at least seven opinions, and this lack of clarity is deeply unhelpful when, as a patient, your clinical knowledge is very limited.

In my experience, particularly given that I have conditions spanning across multiple departments, it has been important to have at least one team acting as a grounding force to guide the direction of treatment. You need a leader who, in your mind, understands the overall picture well enough to advise on the best approach, tailored to you. For me, this has been my hepatologists.

That said, we can't expect doctors to be perfect communicators. Patients often need to do a great deal of administrative legwork – 'synergy' between NHS departments ceased to exist sometime in the 1960s – which isn't ideal when you already have the human equivalent of a four-year-old overheating iPhone's battery capacity. It also helps if patients can learn to talk fluently about their condition. Easier said than done, obviously, but I once had an epiphany during a consultation with a GP that I have, over the years, become an expert in my unique combinations of conditions. It then dawned on me that the only person who knows my own body, its quirks and its variances, is me. But even *I* get it wrong sometimes, so I can't expect doctors to get it right 100% of the time, either.

This leads us to another uncomfortable truth: patients must bear some – arguably *most* – of the responsibility in keeping themselves well, where they are able to. Albeit with the advantage of a background in science, I can recite the quantities and spellings of medications I'm on (having learned the hard way to never trust the NHS to keep this, or my diagnosis list, up to date). I have a sharp recall of all the odd symptoms felt over the last five years, and if the details are hazy, I'll check my meticulously kept diaries, complete with all appointments. I am the weirdo who spends evenings nurturing a curiosity about my condition, going down blue-link paths on Wikipedia, reading research papers and asking ChatGPT why tacrolimus is bad for kidney function. But then again, I have the luxury of time to pore over these things.

With every consultation, the geek in me finds it endlessly interesting to be able to speak to medics who have such specific knowledge about a topic. Entering each consultant appointment armed with a list of things to chat about, I could easily win the award of most irritating patient. Yet I've found that most doctors are all too happy to talk about their area of expertise, to share their knowledge and to educate. Doing so makes them a better doctor, me a much better patient, and the two of us a better team.

I like to think, perhaps arrogantly, that over the last twelve years, my sixth sense for when something is serious has sharpened. Whereas I once freaked out about every twinge, I now have a better sense of the times when I can probably chill out. Bit by bit, I've hopefully become a well-rounded, educated patient who – having been involved in making decisions over the course of months or years – can work with my doctors to keep me healthy for that little bit longer.

*First, do no harm.* The Hippocratic Oath[51] that underpins modern healthcare is, I believe, reflected in almost every interaction I have had with medics. Doctors want to help. Some are better at doing this than others. But most are simply people striving to make the world a better place, and on this one qualification, maybe I could have been a doctor, after all.

[51] Interestingly, 'First, do no harm' (or to be more accurate, the Latin phrase '*primum non nocere*') doesn't actually appear in the Hippocratic Oath, but rather originates from one of Hippocrates' texts called 'Of the Epidemics'. Hippocrates, by the way, was an ancient Greek philosopher/physician who is considered to be the 'father of medicine'. Confusingly, it is thought that he didn't actually write the Hippocratic Oath. Anyways…

# ON FIRST LOVE(S)

There's being a late bloomer in the romance department, and then there's me. If we discount the poster of Leo DiCaprio when I was six, my first kiss was – please don't laugh – aged nineteen. Sadly, like many young girls, my self-confidence plummeted to subterranean depths as a teenager. Throughout school, I deemed myself the least attractive combination of cells imaginable.

It didn't particularly bother me to not have romantic adventures as a teenager because I figured it was generally less disappointing to have crushes on people who I would never meet in real life and therefore had no chance of being rejected by (hello, the cardigan-ed man in the Sugababes' *Push the Button* music video). Besides, I had exams to concentrate on, and my colour-coded mind maps complete with illustrated Appeasement milestones leading to WW2 wouldn't create themselves.

I quite happily plunged a little *too* deeply into my studies, adopting the attitude that I should turn all my attention to bettering my chances of getting into a good university, where I planned to not only get a degree, but also meet the love of my life. I would then move to London, live in a quixotic studio flat like Bridget Jones', buy clothes that were in Grazia magazine, and wear them to an office where I'd chip away at a fulfilling, well-paid and high-flying career in *something.* What exactly I really wanted to do was a moot point.

But then the summer of 2010 dawned. My acne miraculously cleared overnight, and I realised I had quite a nice figure, actually, or at least not awful. I ventured out in bodycon minidresses *without* t-shirts underneath to cover my decolletage[52], began wearing foundation and flaunted a rainbow of BarryM glitter on my eyelids.[53] This new version of me could look in the mirror without wincing and wake up in the morning without panicking about spots she'd have to suffocate with concealer.

The big change was leaving for university, where I had a baptism of fire in meeting so many people from different backgrounds, who were all infinitely smarter, prettier and cooler than me. Learning quickly that having a social life with my newfound pals was a lot of fun, I loved nothing more than getting ready for a night out, cracking out the tunes on YouTube, visiting flats for pre-drinks and card games with rules that I didn't understand, then heading *en masse* to what can only be described as a dungeon masquerading as a nightclub. What's more, Edinburgh had a wider range of good-looking guys than back home in the Highlands.

The problem was that 98% of the boys (and, at 18, they

---

[52] Still kept the opaque tights on, though. Didn't want to be *too* risqué.

[53] Everyone is entitled to a temporary moment of madness.

were still boys, let's face it) I fancied would have had absolutely no idea about it. There was still a massive part of me that lacked enough confidence to flirt, so most of my first two years of university were filled with unrequited crushes. To my embarrassment, most of these crushes were on undeniably attractive but socioeconomically unmatchable '*Hooray Henrys*' who turned up to my Economics 1A tutorials whenever they weren't hungover from ski society benders.

When a boy who I fancied finally showed the merest hint of vague, inebriated interest in me, my heart began loading fuel onto the raging bonfire that was my teenaged imagination. The reality train very quickly went accelerating off the tracks, and whilst I wasn't daft enough to completely lose focus on my studies, the opportunity for romance – something I had only experienced vicariously through novels like *Rebecca* and *Emma* – was too good to pass up.

This was my chance to be the main character in my very own version of a mid-to-late-90s film wherein the sole aim – regardless of career success, friendships, or personal development – was to end up with Hugh Grant. We swapped numbers and chatted on BlackBerry Messenger. When I say 'chatted', I really mean I would send him paragraphs, only to receive a token two sentences in return. But those two sentences provided sufficient textual breadcrumbs to keep me thinking there was *something* there.

Our (and my) first kiss was on the dancefloor during an indie-themed Saturday night at HMV Picturehouse (R.I.P., now a Wetherspoons). Oasis' *Wonderwall,* the theme-track to all of history's great romances which also went on to become my most-played song of 2011, boomed out as we swayed from side to side (albeit out of sync, because my Topshop ballet pumps kept sticking to the tequila-drenched floor).

I tried valiantly over the next few weeks to provide life support to something that never existed in the first place, and after a conversation-less coffee date which I arranged, it was clear this romance was a dead duck. For a relationship which a) never even existed in the true sense of the word, and b) was over in a few weeks, it took me an embarrassingly long time to stop wallowing over him. Playing Adele's *'Someone Like You'* at full blast on my iPod Shuffle, I would find myself ruminating over the 'MERrY XMAS x' text he sent me on the 27th of December (did the kiss mean anything? What was the importance of the small case 'r'? Yes, I was *that* delulu).

I plodded on, moping around on Planet Single for another year, never having really left its atmosphere in the first place, until I met the slightly eccentric but refreshingly *different* (aren't they all?) Dave[54] at a mutual friend's party. He wore a non-tartan shirt which, given it was 2012, was a rare sartorial choice for males under the age of 25. Above all, the fact that secured his green-flag status, accelerating him to pedestal-tier within minutes of our first conversation, was that he used to work in M&S. He had a staff discount card and had saved his mum 40% off her recent sofa. It was meant to be.

I was besotted even before he'd offered me his jacket on the way home. Our first date, some weeks later, was shortly after I had been told I had liver cirrhosis. Every aspect of my life felt like it was tumbling down in freefall: my grandfather was also dying of cancer at the time, I had another lifelong condition to join the lupus and, worse still, was in the middle of a liver flare which wasn't easing despite high doses of steroids. My hair was falling out with the concoction of drugs,

54 Not his real name. There's nothing particularly bad about this story, I'm just trying to keep it a little more coded.

and every day came with a fun new side effect – platelet rashes on my forearms, swollen cheeks, stretch marks over my thighs and my calves and my boobs. My final university exams were a month away, and I had embarked on a low-salt and low-calorie diet in an ill-informed attempt to avoid steroid-induced water retention and weight gain, which made me even more irritable.

I longed so, so much for a snippet of happiness. For *something* to go my way again. For a bit of normality. I felt like I deserved this chance at romance, and I was prepared to ignore the shambles of everything else in my life conspiring against me to get it.

But ignoring everything else became a bit of a problem, and it ultimately meant that I never fully allowed myself to be vulnerable in that relationship. I always tried to be positive, to not honestly talk about my many, many worries. I would always tiptoe around explaining how serious my condition actually was lest I scared Dave away.

"You'll be able to drink again at some point, though, right?" Dave asked over dinner one night, early on in our relationship.

"Yeah. Think so. Not sure when, though," I lied, knowing full well I would never drink a sip again, but keen to keep up appearances of everything being totally cool and totally normal. I didn't want to rock the boat. By doing so, I think it helped me hold on to some kind of normality. If I didn't have that, I could have spiralled to a much darker and lonelier place.

Spending time with him was a fun distraction – I remember visiting London for the first time in my life, him acting as my hipster tour guide round Shoreditch. But ultimately, the difficulty with not being authentic in your closest relationships is that those relationships are then formed on a rather shoogly support base.

Sometimes I felt that Dave was annoyed by my health anxiety; he would say I took things too seriously, or that I needed to relax more. I think these intentions came from a genuinely good place, but they only served to make me feel – time and time again – like I wasn't a good enough girlfriend. I wasn't cool enough, or pretty enough, or healthy enough.

We were both young when we were going out, and whilst he seemed to be the epitome of suave maturity at 23, he really didn't have a clue about much. Neither did I. I can't retrospectively blame him for not supporting me, because I didn't have the skills to communicate how I felt. Fully grown adults in marriages struggle to process chronic illness; to expect us to do this successfully with such little life experience would be unfair.

I think his approach is best summarised in a text he once sent, in response to a text *I* sent to finally explain how upset I was about my hair loss (over text! Text! Why, Kirsty?!). He replied that he would love me even if I had hair like Cheryl Cole, which (I think) perfectly captures the essence of his attempts to be kind.

As time went on, and I began to adjust to life with illness and medical procedures and drugs, I realised that I no longer needed the escape from murkiness. I was able to work through that murkiness on my own, but my relationship with Dave had given me the safe space to practise doing that.

It was overwhelming and brilliant and unrealistic in the way that first loves often are. I'm thankful that I met him when I did, for he brightened my life to offset the gloom that was casting itself over the start of our relationship. I think he means more to me, as my first boyfriend, than I will ever mean to him. Dave, if you ever read this, and you probably won't: I genuinely thank you for being in my life, and for introducing me to Belle and Sebastian.

# ON DATING, SINGLEDOM AND SELF-RESPECT

Grab a coffee and a biscuit. Get comfy. This is going to be a long one.

I once sat through a friend's wedding speech that described how the couple met on what was the groom's *first ever* Tinder match. Cue much hilarity from the audience, and much incredulity from me. On the opposite side of my dining table, another couple turned to each other, eyes wide and mouths agape. The woman leaned in to explain their reaction.

"You won't believe this, but that's exactly how Euan and I met, too! First date on Tinder and – *zing!* – I knew he was the one. So strange, isn't it, how that happens?"

"Uncanny," I replied in a Teuchter drawl, reaching for a flute of warm orange juice to drown my sorrows. Only the previous weekend, I had embarked on my very own six-hundred-and-fourth[55] Tinder date. Needless to say, it was unsuccessful.

I was chuffed to see my friends getting married – they are excellent people who deserve happiness, and it's a lovely reminder that healthy relationships *do* exist in the world – but that didn't stop me from sitting at that table, surrounded by confetti hearts, and reflecting on the dismal state of my own love life.

Having failed to strike gold on the health front, it would be nice if the universe conspired to do me a good turn in the way of romance. I try hard (possibly *too* hard) to be an interesting person; I have hobbies, I exercise, eat healthily, and my job is relatively cool. I enjoy reading and watching films and going to gigs and meeting new people. I reckon I'm a considerate, kind and reasonably 'emotionally intelligent' kinda gal. *Whoo, go me.*

Yet it feels that I never quite reap the dividends of all this effort. While my peers are slowly but surely pairing off, I'm forever left playing the world's smallest violin on this island of singledom.

"And what a great island that could be," my Mum says, trying as she does to make me feel better about everything. "Being able to do what you want, when you want, just for you. A lot of married people would be envious of that, you know."

She's right. Kind of. Being single has many advantages, and whilst it sounds like I'm trying to convince myself through gritted teeth, I am genuinely thankful to have had the freedom to develop into the adult I am today without the influence of,

---

55 604$^{th}$-ish. I don't *literally* keep track.

or the need to consider, anyone except me. I have executive decision over holiday destinations, have painted my bedroom walls pink, and leave dishes unwashed overnight *sans* judgement. I could technically apply to be a beekeeper in the Democratic Congo with no prior consideration of anyone else's life plans.[56]

On reflection, I actually *needed* to be alone in my 20s. Firstly, I was too selfish to be in a proper relationship. But along with that selfishness, I was forced to build myself a support network independently. I had the space to get to grips with my strengths and weaknesses, to date people who were not right for me, and to grow confident in being myself. I learned how to enjoy my own company, navigate round the European train network solo, survive heartbreak (again, and again) and bleed radiators. Generally, I realised I was just about able to handle most situations that life threw at me. That's not to say all of this can't be done in the context of a relationship – it absolutely can – but personally, I needed to stubbornly prove to myself that I could do it all alone first. There is even a small part of me that worries that I would lose some of that self-reliance if I was to be in a relationship.

Yet there's a niggling feeling that my life would have an added dimension if I had a partner with whom to share my experiences and big bags of Tyrrells. I want a partner to support and be supported by, to laugh with and to learn from. Maybe that's overly sentimental, but I think wanting to have a partner with whom to share life's experiences is nothing unusual.

However, *finding* such a partner is proving quite the challenge. I've tried not looking, and I've tried looking. I've

---

[56] Except I wouldn't because of, you know, all the health stuff.

'completed' the apps, and I've sworn myself off the apps. I've signed myself up to every crafting group within a 23 miles radius and now have a spare cupboard rammed full of rusty calligraphy sets. I've gone on 'holiday' to a French language school to meet 'likeminded' people, only to find that the entire class was female. I've done volunteering for community cinemas, climate groups and book festivals, and whilst that's been great fun, I am no further forward in meeting anyone I've clicked with.

Some well-meaning people tell me 'he'll come along soon'. Others advise that it'll happen when I least expect it. These sentiments provide warm fuzzy comfort for all of two microseconds before being frozen by my ice-cold cynicism. I spend most of my time either at work, at the special treatment room having a needle shoved into a vein, or at an outpatient department – three places where I do not expect to find the love of my life. It's unlikely that Prince Charming will burst through the clinic doors yielding a sterilised cannula.

Dating in today's world feels like the antithesis of courtships which generations of old enjoyed. My female forebears never sat on their stools at night, ruminating over what Billy had muttered in their direction at Tuesday's market.[57] Their thumbs were too busy knitting cardigans to be swiping through dating apps, or, as I like to call them, the online purgatory where single people can slowly chip away at their own self-esteem until they reach a point of utter desperation.

I resent pimping myself out on the apps, running through the cyclical failure time and time again. In the years spent flipflopping between Hinge, Tinder and Bumble, there have

[57] One of my grannies was won over by my grandad spilling a box of Maltesers down the stairs at the local cinema; the other pair of grandparents met at a Highland Games. You really couldn't make it up.

been few matches with whom I've pursued more than three dates. Two were lovely blokes who left for jobs at the other side of the country. Another (less lovely) bloke left me stranded halfway up a Munro, suffering from a bout of food poisoning, whilst he proceeded to the summit. One dumped me after three months because *my* health issues gave *him* anxiety, and he thought that *he* worried about me more than *I* worried about me (fair enough, but I assured him that this was not possible). I'm not quite sure which reason hurt the most.

In between, I've had hundreds of dates and chatted to countless more matches. If baseline online dating is as much fun as a toenail extraction, then I can confirm that online dating with a chronic illness is on par with having said extraction performed in a footbath of sulphuric acid.

When I'm slicking liquid eyeliner over my lids before a date, I'm not only praying to Cupid that my match can hold a conversation. I'm also hoping that he doesn't turn up with a viral infection, and that he doesn't notice the impossibly glossy sheen of my fake hair. I'll deliberately wear a long-sleeved top so there's no questions about my forearms being a dot-to-dot of violet-tinged bruises.

Then there's the next hurdle: how best to weave liver disease casually into conversation without red flags being rapidly hoisted? Autoimmune hepatitis doesn't roll off the tongue, and name-dropping cirrhosis (if he knows what it is in the first place) usually causes all sorts of confusion. What to say when he asks why I have the 'no drinking' option selected on my profile? Should I talk about the immunosuppressants? Do I explain I'll likely need a transplant? And if I do, when should I mention all of this? Before dessert, or after? Unpacking an entire medical history into a five-minute cheery lowlights reel is not first date chat fodder. Equally, neglecting to even touch on what is one of the most important aspects of my life feels too much like catfishing.

What if, when I unveil the warts-and-all story, he runs out the restaurant faster than I can feebly mumble, '…but I'm fine, really'? If a date crashes and burns after I reveal my conditions, I attribute the failure to me being 'too much'. And if the date goes well despite me mentioning the liver stuff, then I automatically assume that he didn't fully grasp the seriousness of it all. Dating me is like untwisting an impossible Rubik's cube.

Being diagnosed when I was young means that future partners will never know me without medical compartmentalisation. But then again, it's been so long since even *I've* known that illness-free version of myself. My adult personality today is the sum total of my lived experience, and whilst that's far from being defined entirely by medical issues, it's undeniably influenced by them.

Living with a serious illness is a daunting task, and from time to time I feel like I could be a 'burden' on a partner. Low self-esteem manifests itself in insidious ways, and my insecurities are often brought to the boil whilst dating. Whilst I'm confident in my own ability to deal with my conditions, and have adapted my life accordingly, asking someone else to shoulder this is a step further.

Whilst my parents, sister, friends and ChatGPT all coo in my ear that I'm a lovely person, there's always a poisonous little voice chirruping away on the other shoulder. The voice asking how anyone could love me, with so many things wrong. Asking why anyone would choose to waste time with someone who doesn't know if she'll survive another year, let alone a lifetime. Who would hedge their bets shacking up with someone who they might need to care for? And then the big gun which steamrolls over all other concerns – what if I fall in love with someone, only for them to want children which I cannot have?

Even when I meet someone I like, I catch myself thinking they're too *nice* to get laden with my 'baggage'. I start to self-sabotage, looking for petty reasons why we couldn't possibly work; he likes to share a bottle of wine, perhaps, or he enjoys long-distance hikes which would floor me. It feels unnatural, but I work on reminding myself that I am worthy of a healthy and fulfilling partnership. Life is unpredictable and relationships are, by their very nature, messy. Nobody is problem-free or perfect. To put it bluntly, anyone could get married with textbook good health and get diagnosed with something terminal straight after the honeymoon.

It must be equally challenging to be diagnosed with a serious medical condition whilst in an otherwise stable, long-term relationship. I used to assume that there must be some comfort in knowing that your partner met you *before* illness and would therefore love you unconditionally, in sickness and in health. Having spoken to married people who were diagnosed with illness later in life, I've realised my assumption was Disneyfied. Many feel unsupported by their partners. Indeed, studies have shown that up to 75% of marriages impacted by chronic illness will end in separation.[lxv]

To be honest, I often feel like dating is not really worth the effort. It's mentally exhausting swiping through profiles (and how else do people meet these days?). It's physically exhausting getting psyched to go out and meet someone new. And then there's the actual, very real, health risks; I've never been into sleeping with lots of people out of fear of HPV or herpes, and the inevitable wreckage those viruses (considered relatively minor in otherwise healthy individuals) might have on my fragile ecosystem. Coupled with the fact that sex is often quite painful and results in thrush, UTIs or other infections thanks to immunosuppression, the concept of dating for 'fun' often fades into the ether. This level of analysis is, I'm sure, a lot deeper than what most people bring along to the table on a Tinder date.

To that extent, I've come to view my health conditions as an excellent way to sieve the good guys from the chaff. I can be clear of my (admittedly very high) expectations from the outset of any relationship: I need someone who will be strong enough to support me through some really difficult times, but able to match my dark sense of humour. I don't expect him to name four enzymes produced in the left liver lobe, but rather to understand how to best help me cope with the surprises my body throws out in its own wee medical hoedown.[58] That's quite a lot to ask of someone, and over the years, I've realised that this kind of person is quite rare. But, for reasons I'm not quite sure of, I'm ever hopeful someone like that does actually exist. It might just take me a long time to find him.

For most of my 20s I couldn't shake off the feeling that I *needed* to be dating. I *needed* to be trying to find someone, and not just anyone, but someone I really liked, before I got too ill or too unattractive (this is a very shallow outlook, but it was how I felt). It was as though I thought that once I was in a relationship, that box would be ticked off and my life would fall into place, and everything would be hunky dory. I really wish I could go back and shake some sense into 27-year-old Kirsty, remind her that life doesn't work like that. I'd tell her

---

58 In return, of course, they'll get a loyal partner with a lust for life, who makes personalised birthday cards, takes genuine pleasure from hoovering and whips up pancakes on Sunday mornings *pro bono*.

to chill out. To stay optimistic and enjoy meeting new people, not necessarily for romance but just for the sake of meeting new people. To learn from the process of getting heartbroken, as ridiculous as that concept might seem.

More recently, I've had a wee bit of an epiphany. Whisper it, but I think I've realised that it would be far from the worst eventuality if I never found a partner. Yes, I'll no doubt have nights when I'll wish someone would sit in companiable silence next to me on the sofa. I'll need to watch that I don't become so self-sufficient and headstrong that I close myself off to meeting someone nice.

But ultimately, I know any partner would only add to the rich life I've now built for myself, rather than being the North Star to guide it, as I expected when I was younger. I have a sneaking feeling that the best relationship I'll ever need to be in is the one with myself, and I am determined to enjoy that relationship for as long as I can.

# ON COMPLIMENTS I NEVER REALLY WANTED

1. **Owner of the world's "most palpable spleen".** According to one senior consultant on the ward rounds, mine was the most enlarged spleen he had felt in his entire clinical career. So enlarged, in fact, that he brought over a medical student for a feel, too. In my opinion, go big or go home. In this specific case, I wanted to go big *and* go home; his sign-off was the determining factor as to whether I was well enough to rest back in my own house rather than in hospital. I do have a massive spleen, but not because I've gone to town on chips and cheese. As my liver is now so scarred, it is hard for blood to pass through easily. This causes an increased blood pressure in the veins around the liver and the spleen, creating swelling and pools of blood which then, in turn, enlarge the spleen.
2. **The "most glamorous patient on steroids".** Like a human version of John Lewis, I'm never knowingly underdressed going to medical appointments, and it's

lovely when anybody comments on it. Cosplaying as a minor Royal is a not-so-subtle attempt to convince the wider world – and myself – that I am absolutely, totally fine, totally capable, and totally put together. It is my way of warning people to not pity me: I have a life outside of these hospital doors. I have places to be, and people to see, when I leave this appointment.

3. **Owner of a "remarkably flat stomach".** In the name of transparency, I'll admit that this was only after a month of a strict no chocolate/no sweets/no fun monastic lifestyle during a particularly bad flare of my AIH. My only excuse, you'll understand, for *not* having permanent abs of steel is that fat is generally less painful to cut through than muscle, due to having fewer pain receptors. My thinking (and I have zero scientific proof for this) is that any future liver transplant might then involve less muscle being cut through in my ab region. Therefore I could have reduced recovery times. It's wild and fanciful thinking, but pass me the chocolates anyways.
4. **"Cheeriest patient of the day".** My ego puffed up to bursting point with this one, because part of my inherent people-pleasing is to make everyone else be at ease with my medical misfortune. If I can bring joy to an otherwise joyless bloodletting room, that's a win. In fact, I find it a personal challenge to ramp *up* my happiness levels depending on the medical seriousness of whatever I'm dealing with. It's all an elaborate defence mechanism, of course, but there are worse defences out there.
5. **"Inspirational patient who is a delight".** For context: I wrote a thank you letter to my GP practice during Covid (I truly am a nauseating teacher's pet) and in return was left a lovely voicemail from one of the GPs with this wee accolade. It's a similar tale in clinical

letters where I've been called 'lovely', 'delightful', and 'a pleasure'. These compliments are to be taken with a pinch of salt, as I believe it's medic-code for 'she's compliant, understands the situation and not a complete twit'. Nonetheless, it gives me a little glow.

# ON DRUGS

*"I don't do drugs. I am drugs."*

*Salvador Dali*

Every morning, around 9am, a precise dose of chemicals shoots through my bloodstream. Despite never having smoked a joint, let alone gone within sniffing distance of any illegal pill, powder or popper, I am very reliant on a cocktail of drugs.

I recall a conversation with a consultant about my dose of one particular medicine, called steroids. Over the course of two years, we had been cautiously tapering down my intake, with every eight-month period heralding a paltry milligram's worth of reduction.

"Do you think we'll ever make it to *zero* milligrams? Be off them, you know, completely?" I asked, brimming with hope and enthusiasm and dreams of a non-chubby face.

"That's just not going to happen, I'm afraid."

"Ever?"

"Ever." The doctor scrawled some circles across a bloods order form. "You've been on steroids for so long now that your own adrenal glands probably wouldn't be able to work properly on their own. Plus they're good to have in the background as a maintenance dose, just keeping a dampener on your immune system."

The words fell like a caustic drop of vinegar onto my wounds of unobtainable perfectionism, but the reality is that my body can't sustainably look after itself. If my cells don't get their fix of immunosuppression, my nervous system enters a state of withdrawal, with potentially fatal consequences. This dependence niggles away in my mind more than it probably should. For whilst my drugs are regulated, and are made in a QC-checked laboratory, having passed all the relevant data trials, there is something of a parallel to be drawn between my reliance on drugs and that of someone facing addictions of another, more nefarious, kind. At the end of the day, we are both victims of circumstance, dealing with situations which nobody wants to find themselves facing.

The irony is not lost on me that, pre-diagnosis, my lifetime's number of prescriptions was in single figures. Whereas I used to refuse paracetamol unless my pain was intolerable, today I'm the only one of my friends known to have taken fentanyl straight in the veins. But shifting from puritanical abstainer to daily pill-popper takes adjustment, and this transition was considerably easier when I started to properly understand *why* these drugs were necessary.

So here begins a whistlestop tour of three pharmacological wonders doing the heavy lifting required to keep my body – and that of so many others with autoimmune conditions – going.

**Prednisolone**

First off, we have *la crème de la crème* of the pharmacological tool kit: the mighty steroid. Known the world over for all the wrong reasons, steroids are medicine's answer to the notorious Kray twins. There's the utter nutcase (the anabolic steroid) and its more conscientious (but equally depraved) brother, the corticosteroid.

***Anabolic*** steroids are Class C drugs, legal only for personal use, not supply or sale. They are often misused by beefcake poseurs who spend more time admiring themselves in the gym mirrors than actually using gym machines. Anabolic steroid use comes with a list of side effects more protracted than Lance Armstrong's count of doping offences, but we're not going to spend time on them.

***Cortico*****steroids,** the bread and butter of many autoimmune disease medicine regimes, are the pharmaceutical equivalent of the fire brigade. An emergency call to corticosteroids will potentially involve an intravenous treatment to extinguish inflammation in a matter of hours.

There are topical formulations for skin aggravations, whilst asthmatics can take the steroids via an inhaler to the lungs. They are quite literally lifesaving for other people too – facilitating cancer treatments and preventing Crohn's attacks to name but two of their alternative indications.[59]

[59] Fancy word for conditions that can be treated using the drug.

My specific corticosteroid, called ***prednisolone***, comes in the form of little white pills that, should you ever have the misfortune of having one stuck on your tongue, leave an aftertaste resembling a shot of Fairy liquid laced with battery acid. Prednisolone breaks out of the blister foils like a knight in shining armour and rides into my bloodstream on his mighty steed, putting a damp towel over the smouldering bushfire that is my overactive immune system.

Keen to provide a balanced view, I'll present the positives of steroids. They're cheap, they're well-studied, and they pack a powerful punch. Bottom line, they help keep my flares at bay and therefore help keep me alive. At high doses (which are normally given in the short-term due to the drug's potency), they give me so much energy that I feel capable of single-handedly reversing climate change whilst negotiating peace talks with Pyongyang. My thought process revs up to the extent that I need to make a conscious effort to slow the internal monologue.

Thing is, in the longer term, Prince Prednisolone becomes a royal pain in the arse. Reading the patient information leaflet will leave even the most upbeat patient wanting to curl up into a ball, questioning whether the rest of life is worth living if it means waiting for the plague of possible adverse effects to arrive at their house.

High-dose prednisolone can cause mood swings to rival extreme PMS, and those innocuous white pills have been known to fill me with an inexplicable sense of dread. A minor inconvenience – realising that there is no milk left in the fridge for a cup of tea, as a purely hypothetical example which definitely has not happened – could, under the influence of steroids, be viewed as the biggest problem ever faced by mankind, giving way to 15 minutes of snotty tears.

Some people suffer more serious psychological side effects, such as steroid-induced psychosis or depression. Indeed, during my first rodeo on steroids I realised quite how terrifying it is to not feel in total control of your own mental health. My brain felt unfamiliar; my thoughts tainted with the chemical makeup of the steroids and their impact on my hormones.

Steroids often make people want to eat everything within a five-mile radius, though I often *lose* my appetite with high doses. They make my tastebuds tinge with metal, as though I have a spoon pressed against my tongue all the time. Headaches, nausea, and diarrhoea are also par for the course. And then we have the delightful 'moonface': steroids mess up the bodily distribution of fat, meaning that long-term steroid use can cause fat to migrate to the facial cheeks and neck. They also cause fluid retention which doesn't help the bloating, either. Finally, steroids can also cause an overproduction of cortisol, which can further contribute to a bloated face.

It's a long and protracted process to wean off prednisolone, and the taper down can't be done too quickly. Tapering off steroids is often the hardest part, with more headaches, nausea, shakiness and other withdrawal symptoms. Sometimes the taper can't ever happen. In this case, you're wedded to steroids for the (life)long haul.

And this is where the nastiness of steroids really comes into its own. Long-term steroid use increases the risk of developing: osteoporosis (bone thinning and propensity for breakages), diabetes, eye problems, insomnia, difficulty with skin healing, cardiac problems, weight gain, hormonal insufficiency, pretty much any cancer but especially skin cancers, reduced ability to clear viruses which infect skin cells (such as HPV), blood clotting issues, susceptibility to infection, and more serious complications from these infections. Then there are the niche spin-off conditions that steroids can contribute towards, such as hip necrosis (as mentioned in my opening chapter) and probably another 10,000 conditions I'll never know about. The list goes on and on. These drugs are amazing, but they're brutal.

Taking medication for a chronic illness is a lifelong game of whack-a-mole; trying to thump down the initial problem only ends up causing ten more to spring up elsewhere in the system. Over time, the side effects of the original medication will end up needing to be medicated, too. *Aegrescit medendo*, as the philosopher Virgil once said[60]: *the cure is worse than the disease.* Which is why, then, the best medicine is prevention. Medicine can only help us so far, and I'm afraid too few people understand that before it becomes too late. We need to help ourselves in the first instance by leading healthy lives. Youth is wasted on the young, and health is wasted on the healthy.

**Tacrolimus**

Visiting Japan is on my bucket list, but my cheapest quote for worldwide travel insurance exceeds three grand. So instead of downing matcha in a tea ceremony, I make do with downing ***tacrolimus***, a drug that was discovered at the University of Tokyo back in the 1980s.

The research group set out to find an immunosuppressant for transplant patients which didn't destroy the bone marrow to the same extent as some of the others available at the time. They ended up with a fermented broth of a soil sample from

---

60 Apparently. Though it's also been attributed to Francis Bacon and Albert Einstein, so who really knows? The Latin makes it sound fancier.

a mountain 60km northeast of Tokyo, called Mount Tsukuba. This broth contained the bacteria *Streptomyces tsukubaensis*[lxvi], which produces the immunosuppressant tacrolimus (***T***sukuba m***acrol***ide ***im***m***u***no***s***uppressant).[lxvii]

To add to the excitement, there are various forms of tacrolimus, all with equally confusing names. And, unhelpfully, they are all non-interchangeable; if I'm on one version of tacrolimus, I cannot just simply swap over to the same dosage of a different version of tacrolimus. The swap must be done under careful monitoring. So, if I end up at the hospital, I pray to the pharmacy gods that they've both got my brand of tacrolimus in stock and got the most updated notes on their systems, to ensure the right version is prescribed (and, from experience, I never assume this happens automatically).

Approved in Japan in 1991 for liver transplantation patients, tacrolimus works to ensure that the body's immune system doesn't spot the massive elephant in the room that is a different person's organ having been swapped in. The thing with tacrolimus is that whilst it's a great immunosuppressant, it's also poisonous. Here are the two 'safety symbols' for tacrolimus on PubChem[lxviii], the repository with deep-dive intel about every chemical known to mankind:

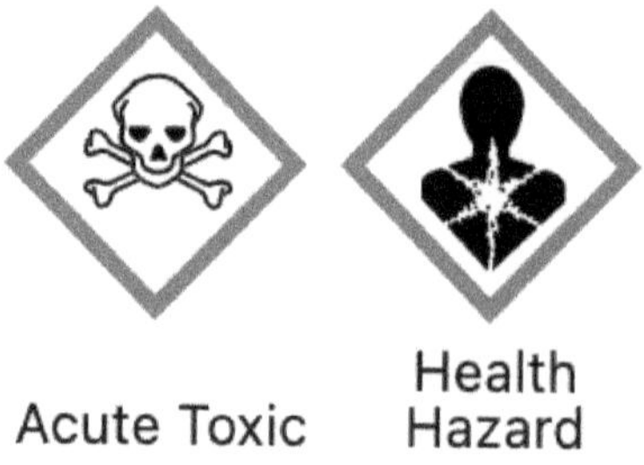


It doesn't take a PhD-level chemist to guess that a bright red pointy diamond around a skull and crossbones is not giving 'wellness vibes'. Indeed, tacrolimus is a dab hand at damaging kidneys, and it doesn't even have the courtesy to selectively destroy one of them at a time. As it's a tricky chemical for the kidneys to filter out of the bloodstream, over the long term, it can cause slow-burn kidney failure.

Tacrolimus, which has a direct impact on the neurological (nerve) pathways in the body, can cause *neurotoxicity*. Symptoms of this range from mild tremors (sometimes transplant patients have shaky hands if you watch closely) through to seizures or full-blown brain damage. I once had a severe headache (possibly the most pain I've ever been in) and was taken to hospital, where we learned that tacrolimus levels in my bloodstream were roughly double what they should have been. My migraine and vomiting were due to burgeoning neurotoxicity. The body's ability to not-so-subtly flash the hazard lights never ceases to amaze me; it's often a matter of hoping doctors can figure out the mystery before a nuclear meltdown.

Tacrolimus is quite the Mariah Carey of my medical box. Its diva demands include needing to be taken at the same time every second day, with copious amounts of water. However, it needs to be stored far away from water at all other times, and always kept at temperatures below 25°C, but above freezing. It must be taken either two hours after, or one hour before, food…and under no circumstances can tacrolimus be taken at the same time as any substance containing the CYP3A4 enzyme (found in marmalade and grapefruit juice, so not a massive inconvenience). In fact, even transplant departments in different hospitals have variations in their guidelines for the approved list of food and drink with tacrolimus.

**Carvedilol**

I like the name of this one, because it's short and snappy –

a drug rep's marketing dream – and somewhat easier to spell out to the GP receptionist on the phone than others (here's looking at you, *hydroxychloroquine*). I especially like the 'lol' at the end, because it's the only thing remotely funny about this drug.[61]

Carvedilol is a type of drug called a beta-blocker, and it's the closest I'll ever come to a legal high. Thing is, it doesn't even make me high. On the converse, it chills me out a bit. Designed to reduce blood pressure, I do sometimes think carvedilol prevents my heart rate rising anywhere above a gentle canter.

Why is it so important that my blood pressure doesn't turn into the bodily equivalent of an EDM bassline? Well, high-blood pressure overall means that there will also be high blood pressure in the plumbing that goes in and out of my liver. *That* plumbing is already pressurised due to my liver itself being a tough old boot, so the blood can't flow through all that easily. Carvedilol is a bit like a preventative measure to lessen the likelihood of the swollen bits in my portal vein spontaneously bleeding.

Of all my drugs, carvedilol is the one I most liken to a politician. It's all talk, and very little action. Put it this way, I wouldn't trust lending carvedilol a fiver. I've taken it since I was 19 yet still suffered a bleed in my mid-20s and have needed numerous banding procedures over the years to re-eliminate swollen varices. Arguably, carvedilol's mechanism is not a watertight preventative measure in my body. That said, research shows that carvedilol might have the additional bonus of reducing the risk of decompensation in patients, so I'll keep taking it for now.

---

[61] Beta-blockers commonly end in the suffix 'lol'. They are designed to lower blood pressure.

Perhaps I appear too flippant about taking heavy-duty medication. Believe me, I'm more than aware of their toxicity. Every morning, when I bunch what are essentially low-dose chemotherapy drugs into my gob, I'm reminded of the fact I'm poisoning myself, albeit in a roundabout way.

But I am fully cognisant of the benefits and remain laser-focussed on the hard truth that taking these drugs is simply the least-bad scenario. I'm relieved, in some ways, that treatment exists, because many diseases don't have this option. Unfortunately, it's an almost guaranteed rule that the more chronic or life-threatening the condition, the more militant the army of combatant drugs – and their side effects – will be. The risk-benefit ratio becomes a little starker and the stakes a little higher. If I don't take them, my overall health would depreciate fast. When faced with the options of either taking a drug that will damage an organ slowly, or not taking it and have another organ damaged a hell of a lot *faster*, my decision is not made any more palatable but is simplified: chin up and chug down.

The most bewildering bit is that when you're diagnosed with chronic disease, you don't have a great deal of time to accept this change to your hitherto-held world view. Instead, one day you visit a doctor and are told that you're now reliant on these serious medicines for life. That's when you're chucked over the audience safety barriers into the Gladiator lion pit, where you'll soon find yourself fighting for survival against not only the original illness snapping at your heels, but also against the raft of side effects conspiring against you. *Are you not entertained?*

I remember telling my boss at a summer café job about my (what was then newly diagnosed) liver condition. I said I was on immunosuppressants. He screwed up his face. "Well, make sure they don't give you too much of that shit, because that's what poisoned my brother. He died from cancer," he replied whilst slicing down a little too hard through an onion on the chopping board. I was grateful for the onion vapour in the room because it disguised the tears that were already in my eyes. I take these drugs because I need to, and it's bloody scary enough without everyone else's opinion in the mix.

The thing is, usually 'everyone else' has a warped idea of the capability of pharmaceuticals, because medicine lulls us, Hansel and Gretel-style, into a false sense of security with all its dazzlingly impressive advances. Sensationalist media loves nothing more than hyping up a new "wonder drug" which will be the panacea to all of society's ills. *Cancer?* Here, try one of these shiny new immunotherapies. *Heart palpitations?* Grab yourself some statins along with your fake tan next time you're in Boots. We sleep soundly, satisfied with our tacit understanding that the humans clever enough to put man on the moon must also be smart enough to have a solution for disease when it falls upon our doorstep. Most of us don't dare question that belief until we must face up to it in the form of a serious diagnosis.

Pharmacological understanding is advancing at a miraculous rate – great news all round for those of us who are ill – but there is still one heck of a lot of gaps in our collective medical understanding. Whilst experts have nailed down a lot of the fundamentals, there are still massive therapeutic areas (cough, cough – *autoimmunity* and *women's health*) of which we are only beginning to prod beneath the surface. Often, I think that the more we learn about the body, the more we realise we just don't know much about it at all.

It's all very well pontificating about this, but it's unsettling and often very alienating to be sat on the receiving end of this uncertainty as a patient. The drugs I take *seem* to work, and are evidence-based, but doctors often admit to only understanding the pharmacology behind the mode of action *to an extent*. "We're not quite sure why that's working,", or "we're not quite sure why that's *not* working' are both phrases I've heard more times than I would ideally want to.

What happens when they don't work for you, or when you're max-ed out on the highest available dose but the response is as effective as stemming an arterial blood loss with Kleenex? Or when you experience side effects akin to being on a week-long bender with the Rolling Stones circa 1970s, that nobody else seems to get? In my experience, for example, steroids don't reduce inflammation quite as fast as they should. It's often a delay of several weeks before my liver function numbers begin a downward trajectory. Side effects can be withstood if it feels like there is a means to an end. But when patients persevere through hair loss and vomiting and losing breasts or wombs, only for the therapies to not achieve the goal, then the output is altogether more devastating. You end up with all the cost, and none of the benefit: a double whammy of disappointment.

In fact, you can't focus on that aspect too much because you're worried instead about what delightful 'next line' concoction you'll be taking next. Often, this will be a drug that is second choice for good reason – either it's not normally as effective, or it has worse side effects. It's like a really shite tombola, where each prize is as bad as the last, but you hope that at least one of them will work in the end – because if not, then you're up the creek without a paddle.

As much as chemists try to build in risk mitigation with research and regulations, at the end of the day, the long-term stage of any clinical trial is essentially – *whisper it* – when it's taken by the wider population and monitored for adverse effects. Even then, nobody will have taken my drugs with quite the same dynamics and conditions and diet and metabolism as me before. As much as the medicines may be deemed safe for use within the laws of clinical trials, I'm all too aware that I'm still a rather glamorous guinea pig.

The sad truth is that unless there are mind-blowingly huge scientific advances, there will be no point in time in my life when I'll stop being a guinea pig. Even if the drugs continue to work, there's a gnawing frustration, a lack of control, over not having an endpoint of these medications. This dependency drives a cold stake into the heart of a control freak.

When I was first put on steroids, I dealt with the lack of control in the only way I knew how: by meticulously planning it. I ripped out an A4 piece of paper from my notepad and started sketching out a 'tapering schedule'. Each week would entail a reduction of 5mg, which meant that within seven weeks I would be completely clear of prednisolone. Of course, what I didn't realise was that nothing – *nothing* – works to plan like this in real life. Thus, 49 days eventually turned into 13 years (and counting) of being on steroids.

I will die if my medicines aren't made, and whilst there's no amount of cuddles or kind words that will change the compulsion to scream into a dark void when that realisation takes hold of my thoughts, I take comfort in knowing that there are millions of other people in a similar boat. I focus on today and take things as they come.

With all the emotional turmoil built into taking prescribed medication, it never ceases to amaze me that people take illegal drugs for pleasure.[62] Each to their own and all that, but knowing quite how many ways in which the body can go easily and completely wrong, I wouldn't want to risk messing that up for the sake of a bit of fun. Secondly, I've never been in a party where I've felt a need to spin round to my pal and say, "You know what I feel would really be the cherry atop of this cake? Some crack cocaine." Maybe I had low expectations of nights out, but back when I used to go to nightclubs, I would be quite easily transported to drug-like euphoria if the DJ played *Mr Brightside*.

Having worked for pharmaceutical and medical device companies, I have seen first-hand the levels of research, development, validation, cleaning protocols, and quality control that ensure that every single dose of that pill, lotion or vaccine is made safely. Even prior to all this medical stuff going on in my life, I was never tempted to verge into drugs because not only was I too scared, but I also had absolutely no idea where I would even go about getting them. Ordering from the Argos catalogue was the extent of my procurement abilities as a teenager.

The explosion of social media now means we are #blessed with ill-informed influencers. I have seen adverts for fertility/weight loss/hair loss advice pushed by the Instagram Illuminati whose closest encounter with a medical textbook was walking past the non-fiction in Waterstones en route to Mills and Boon.

Perhaps my cynicism is unfair. There are people on social media who genuinely think that they are helping people by pooh-poohing 'western medicine'. I've already set out that modern medicine is by no means a cure-all. Equally, papaya

---

[62] To be clear, what I discuss here is recreational drug use, not drug addiction.

smoothies are not likely to rid you of tuberculosis, and yoga at 9pm every Thursday is not going to magically increase your egg count. At best, their advice will do no harm, but if we (i.e. Governments) continue facilitating social media to be a fertile breeding ground for unverifiable, unregulated advice with no accountability, then we risk catapulting ourselves back to the Dark Ages. We need to re-establish that social contract of trust in medical experts: the doctors, nurses, researchers, and professors who study science for years.

What really grinds my gears is the antivax movement and how much traction this ideology continues to get thanks to the online printing press. I will never understand the argument that vaccines are a way to control society, but then again, I always forget that Edward Jenner's work on smallpox was all just a precursor to prepare Bill Gates for worldwide domination. The double standards make me laugh: how some people will decry prescription medication or vaccines because of all the 'chemicals', but have no qualms taking illegal drugs (cut up with who knows what), smoking tobacco (proven to be carcinogenic), vaping (with its questionable safety profile) or polishing down their bathrooms in a viral TikTok video using sodium hypochlorite dissolved in uric acid (a.k.a. bleach).

It's incredible, too, how many shamans drop their long-held moral philosophies like hot potatoes when it comes to accepting treatments for illnesses that can't simply be cured by extra Vitamin C. Anti-vaxxers often renege quietly on their taglines when faced with terminal diagnoses, and all but the most fervent gratefully accept the treatment that drug companies, against whom they've spent years protesting, have developed in the meantime.

There is a special place in hell reserved for any soul who dares convince me that, by swapping my medications for sipping a 40mg spinach wheatgrass blend, my scarred liver will be healed. I also don't appreciate being told that *I* am the cause of my own condition, or that if I'd just been a little less stressed (or had eaten more fish, or less chicken, or not been near Wifi, or had refused the HPV vaccine when I was 15 years old…) that my immune system would be a-okay.

I recall one afternoon in the consulting room with my gastroenterologist, discussing my first round of steroids. They weren't working in quite the way we expected them to.

"Medicine, I'm afraid," he shifted a little uncomfortably in his chair, "is often less of a science, and more of an *art*."

I refrained from replying that if that was the case, then my prescription script was distinctly Pollok-esque. My coping mechanism these days is simply to not think too much about the drugs I take. I accept there's science behind them, but it's not always neatly contained within colour-in lines. It's a bitter pill to swallow, but it's one that must still be swallowed, nonetheless.

# ON TRUSTING THE PROCESS

The first rule of Invisalign[63] Club is that nobody admits to being in Invisalign Club. After all, you've forked out a substantial amount of money for orthodontic braces that are specifically designed to be, well, *invisible*. But it's so secretive that it becomes difficult to find fellow Invisalign-ers to ask questions about the whole experience. This is how I ended up making the grave error of firstly searching for, and then latterly joining, a couple of Invisalign Reddit threads.

If there's one rule for life, it's that it is best enjoyed without joining any Reddit threads, because they have a disconcerting propensity to suck you into black holes of blind, keep-you-up-at-night levels of panic about things that you didn't even know you needed to think about. Whilst the Invisalign community veered towards the better (i.e. less tinfoil hat) end of the Reddit spectrum, it's probably not worth a visit unless you enjoy flipping through photos of misaligned canines and actively wish to waste precious moments of life learning about how

[63] For those not in the know, Invisalign is a clear dental brace.

turmeric reacts with the retainers' plastic and turns them green.

The Invisalign strategy, for those unfamiliar with orthodontal straightening, is that the teeth shift in minor movements over many weeks. Invisalign-ers must accept that there may well be weeks where little visible progress is made. There may even be weeks where a tooth looks less aligned than before. But ultimately, as the religious Redditors would repeat *ad nauseum*, this was all normal. "Trust the process" was a key mantra rolled out, time and time again, on the thread.

Why is teethgeek34's retainer on week 7 not fitting properly? *Trust the process.* Will tonyb1923 need further refinements? *Trust the process.* Is this premolar slightly out of line for where it should be according to orthoque3n's 3D scan? *Trust. The. Process.* Some people put a little too much trust in the process, clinging onto the belief that one more plastic retainer was all that came between them and a face like Angelina Jolie.

Nonetheless, I liked the mantra's three-word snappiness, and reasoned it had application to other elements of life, too. Which is why I now find myself chanting when I'm in a medical pickle: *Trust the process. Trust the body. Trust the medicine.*

When you're so used to being told that you are 'non-textbook' or that things are going wrong in your body, it's tricky to buy back into the idea that it can work as it should. Before long, you find yourself holding more faith in astrology predictions than in the body's abilities to function normally. My (not very healthy) strategy for accepting how many medical problems I have is to adopt a mindset wherein I automatically assume that more bits of me are going to go haywire at any juncture and then be pleasantly surprised when they don't.

Diagnoses, whether scattergun-ed over an intense few days or drip-fed one after another over months and years, force you to pull into question what you thought you innately knew about how your body works. For me, being diagnosed with chronic illness involved a sickening realisation that I didn't really understand how things work at all. My body just *worked,* and then one day it suddenly didn't. The result was a fairly hefty loss of confidence.

Yet despite how difficult and unlikely it may seem, it is possible to maintain some degree of faith in human biology and in the body's ability to heal itself. Where there is life, there is hope. I've been proved wrong time and time again when my body actually does (gasp!) *the right thing.* For example, the time when my kidney function improved when I reduced the dose of a particular drug. Or the time when my cervix miraculously cleared itself of HPV after 12 years of abnormal smear tests. Even when mystery IBS-type symptoms that plagued me for two years cleared up almost overnight. The fact that my body has managed to work round having a cirrhotic liver for a decade is testament to trusting my body to just get on with surviving.

My 'trust in the process' extends beyond pure hardcore science, too. Without wanting to sound *delulu* – I'm not suggesting we all stop our meds and just have blind faith that our bodies will do the right thing – I often wonder if, in the grander scope of the universe, things are operating at an unexplainable, subconscious level. For example, I had my internal bleed a day prior to the start of what should have been a holiday to Copenhagen, thus avoiding being ill abroad (and vomiting blood on a plane, which remains one of my worst fears). A less extreme version would be when I forget to take my medicines in the morning. Five minutes into my commute, I'll be struck with a random train of thought which will eventually remind me that I've not swallowed my daily dose.

Coincidence? Perhaps. Or did my body just *know*? Either way, it provides me with comfort to know that my body is remarkably resilient. The human survival instinct runs deep, and in ways we can't quite fully comprehend. We maybe need to trust it a wee bit more often.

# ON 29[64] THINGS I FEEL BAD ABOUT

1. Sometimes not being in the mood to chat about the weather to the nurse who is taking my bloods, or not really wanting to divulge my 'story' for the umpteenth time to new ultrasound technicians. I know I have the right not to, but I feel compelled to be *nice.* Then I feel bad for being a people-pleaser.
2. Using fancy words like 'neutropenic' and 'immunocompromised' on the phone to the GP receptionist to emphasise the importance of why I need to speak to a doctor, and then having to spell the words out for them to write on my notes. I feel like a pretentious and demanding twit.
3. Being jealous of other people's good health.
4. Not being able to attend a friend's (outdoor) hen do towards the end of the pandemic because I was still scared of crowds.

---

[64] IL-29 is a protein in the body which helps the immune system. Recent research suggests that IL-29 dysfunction has a key role to play in some autoimmune conditions. Hence, I've settled on 29 things.

5. That speeding ticket in 2019 (63 in a 60, seeing as you asked).
6. Being healthier, and having more energy, than a lot of people with my conditions.
7. Missing another friend's wedding breakfast because I had insane IBS and was heavily reliant on Imodium just to make it into the bridesmaid photo.
8. Taking time off work for medical appointments.
9. The inequality in that I am lucky enough to have access to free medical treatment when a great portion of the world does not.
10. Questioning doctors' opinions too much.
11. Not questioning doctors' opinions enough.
12. Bailing on social events because I feel unwell.
13. Ghosting people on dating apps because they have too many pictures with alcohol or can't use apostrophes.
14. Not meeting the love of my life aged 18 and marrying him and therefore reducing my risk of getting HPV by only having one sexual partner, ever. HPV is the bane of my life, because it doesn't always just 'clear after a few months' in immunosuppressed people. It can linger for years and cause lots of problems, but they don't tell you *that* in the sex ed classes.
15. Feeling sorry for myself.
16. Inwardly telling people to piss off when they're constantly moaning about things that are really, in the grand scheme of things, inconsequential.
17. Being a bitch to those closest to me when I'm upset or annoyed, because I've used up all my nice vibes on everyone else.
18. Knowing that, in generations to come, people with my conditions will have to face the impacts of climate change alongside the impacts of chronic illness.
19. Following on from (18), the environmental impact of all the plastic waste from tourniquets, wigs, plasters, pill

packets, needles and blood tubes that are used to treat me.

20. Being too judgemental about everything and everyone.
21. Using up so many consultants' time across more or less every department in the NHS.
22. Taking more from the state system than I will ever contribute, even though I fundamentally believe that healthcare should be a universal right.
23. My habit of sometimes making everything about me in family discussions.
24. Pushing people away sometimes when I don't necessarily *want* to, simply because I think it will be better for everyone if I self-contain my sadness.
25. Not being able to make my mum and dad grandparents.
26. Having too high expectations and then being disappointed when reality doesn't match them.
27. Sometimes feeling hatred towards my body for not working as it should, when I know I should be appreciative of how, despite being so ill, it allows me to live a full life.
28. Putting my family through the stress of watching me be ill, and all that comes with that. In some ways, I think it's easier to have the control of going through the situation myself rather than be a helpless parent or sibling watching the car crash unfold.
29. My cankles.

# ON BEAUTY

Life in the Scottish Highlands leads to a blissful ignorance, should you wish to adopt it, of beauty trends. My makeup routine takes all of three minutes: moisturiser, SPF, concealer slapped on like tribal war paint, mineral foundation that creeps into my mini-wrinkles, eyebrow pencil, blush, then mascara. I've yet to foray into the world of contouring because it frightens me in the same way that panic takes hold whenever I stumble mistakenly into the weights area of a gym. From time to time, I'll catch wind of a new fad online that only serves to confirm quite how much of a sheltered life I lead.

You can imagine my horror, then, when I read an article about a new craze sweeping over Hollywood: *buccal fat removal.* For those unacquainted with this latest Draconian attempt to make women feel inadequate, I'll explain: essentially, the fatty pad in the cheek – the bit we need to smile, that gives us the look of a healthy human being – is surgically sucked out. Why would anyone want to do this? Besides lining the pocket of some depraved cosmetic surgeon, buccal fat removal aims to 'enhance' the jawline, 'emphasise' the cheekbones, and 'improve' facial structure. The thought did occur to me that this could be a perfect way to get rid of prednisolone moon face. Begone, chubby cheeks! Conspire to reveal the razor-sharp cheekbones again!

The extent to which people go to be more 'beautiful' never fails to surprise me. Regardless of the immediate output, I couldn't help but wonder: what are the longer-term effects of buccal fat removal? Our bodies have fat in those cheeks for a reason, and it's a dangerous game to start playing with what nature intended. What about when the collagen naturally wastes away from the face? Will these women (and men) then be queueing up for buccal fat *implants*?

Of course, celebrities operate under different rules of engagement than us mere mortals; rightly or wrongly, it's usually part of their job description to look good. But what remains the preserve of the American elite today, runs the risk of becoming acceptable (or even expected) for average Joannas the world over in a few years' time. It's more than a wee bit disconcerting to herald in yet another way we can change our appearance to align with societal expectations, rather than just being ourselves.

Whilst celebrities have always offered an unachievable beauty standard, we all sort of *know* that they have surgeries and filters and veneers and airbrushing and personal chefs. The big shift, I think, is that social media has now somehow managed to plonk those unrealistic standards on a rocket hurtling at the speed of light towards the general public. No judgement on anyone who does get surgical enhancements – your body, your choice – but I'll provide my take on it.

Swathes of us pore over "get ready with me" reels, watching

influencers brandish the latest must-have false eyelashes, and spout off about the top ten things to eat in order to avoid – heaven forbid! – bloating. Instagram channels are dedicated to salmon-sperm creams to reduce wrinkles whilst unqualified ingénues blabber on YouTube about how kale leaves stuffed inside the vagina will banish yeast. These same influencers whisper the word 'chemical' as if by its mere mention, it will invoke three different types of cancer, ignoring the unsexy truth that our entire universe is filled with nothing other than chemicals.

Nonetheless, the hoops to jump through to be considered pretty are growing ever more complex and conflicting. By constantly redefining what it means to be beautiful, we are simply setting ourselves and future generations up for failure, whilst forgetting that the only real winner is capitalism, magicking up a solution to every insecurity for a very pretty price.

And this all makes me very sad, because chronic illness has changed my outlook on what beauty means. It has flagged the true importance of my body's functions, taught me about the bread and butter of its inner workings. Being ill has required my body to be put through some tough challenges, to garner a strength that it might not have ever needed before. Through this, a level of self-assurance is obtained.

Even when I was a teenager, I never once considered myself pretty, and illness has undoubtedly made me feel even less physically attractive. Every time I look in the mirror, I'm reminded of my disease, that my body is struggling to keep the charade going. My inner critic heads straight for the liver disease bloat underneath my boobs and the steroid bloat in my face, the purple pools under my eyes, the ever-present shiny head with threadbare hair, the broken thread veins peppered across my nose and lash line and lip line, the unexplained bruises that appear on my arms and ankles and neck, the varicose veins on my legs, the burst blood vessels in the dulled whites of my eyes, the tiny warts scattered on my forehead, the thinning eyebrows, the red palms, and the cysts on my shoulder blade. I don't say all this to garner sympathy, or to beckon coos of 'oh, but Kirsty, nobody notices'. It's just how I see myself.

Sure, I can cover a lot of it up with makeup and wigs, so people don't notice. But *I* notice. *I* know it is all just an illusion. It's not the real me; it's the version that I paint on to face the world, because I care too much about what I look like. Nobody is forcing me to, of course. It's my own decision and it makes me feel better. With my makeup and hair, I feel more alive, more healthy, but not necessarily more authentically *me.*

There are times I've looked at myself barefaced and thought: *holy macaroni, I'm in my 30s but look like a frail, washed-out pensioner.* Yet somehow, whilst I don't find my natural, make-up-free reflection pretty, I equally don't find it ugly. Only the people I'm very close to get to see that side of me, and in a strange way, that makes it a bit special.

I actually view it with something of admiration, because I'm very proud of my body for keeping me alive. To have experienced, time and time again, living in states of heightened vulnerability, and to have worked through it with (I like to think) something resembling positivity and grace, is a different and more long-lasting version of beauty.

I sometimes hear women say that the upside of growing older is that they're more 'at peace' with their bodies; they no longer feel some kind of pressure to conform to beauty standards, or to look a certain way for the male gaze or otherwise. They feel freer to just not give a damn. Chronic illness has liberated me in a similar fashion.

I don't consider myself to be in direct competition with the young nubile ladies with their clean bills of health, because I know now that I'm on my own track. Do I still feel jealous of women with naturally great bone structure, good hair and toned bodies? Yes. Would I feel quite so puritanical if wigs didn't exist, or if Natural Collection decided they were stopping production of the only concealer which hides my thread veins? No. Do I look at my perennially bruised legs and pushed-out stomach and wish I didn't have cirrhosis? Often. I'm human. I want to look good. I just don't beat myself up too much for not meeting an expectation which I'll never be able to meet. It would have been nicer, of course, if I had reached this realisation without autoimmune disease needing to bring me there.

Even if I did have a moment of madness and decide to sign up for buccal fat removal, I'd be setting off alarms from all angles. Firstly, my immunosuppression means the risk of infection would be too high for any surgery that wasn't essential. Then there would be the possible contraindication of whatever anaesthetics or injectables used reacting with the medicines I take, or even triggering an autoimmune response. Lastly, any kind of medical intervention carries risks of complications (excessive bleeding, for one, would not be great with my low platelet count). It's a no-brainer to me that having razor-sharp cheekbones would never justify the risk of surgery going wrong.

It's all fine and well me chatting about this as a 30-something. I imagine it's tough getting older, but as someone who doesn't have a guaranteed future[65], I can't help but see ageing as anything other than a privilege. I'd be honoured to have wee wrinkles etched in my face and smile lines at the corner of my mouth, because the alternative is that I don't make it to the age where I can do this. That, to me, is a much sadder outcome.

The boring truth is that, often, the best beauty advice has been doing the rounds for decades and costs next to nothing. But nobody is going to get paid on Instagram for extolling the virtues of a vegetable-filled diet, with no drinking, no smoking, moderate exercise, and ample sleep.

Illness has no room for vanity and will happily deplete 'attractiveness' for the sake of staying alive, but it also strips back the concealers and reveals the human body for the beautiful machine that it is. There isn't anything quite as adaptable or wonderfully complex as the getup we walk around in every day. That should be justification in itself for why every one of us deserves self-love. We shouldn't feel the need to surgically modify that body to meet some passing trend, or punish it, or deny it food and nutrients. All I wish for is that we all could learn to accept our bodies as they are and give them the due love and respect they so deserve.

[65] Though none of us do, really, do we?

# ON (NOT) ACHIEVING EXPECTATIONS

Dopamine is one hell of a drug. Picture the scene: a school classroom full of nine-year-olds, jostling over each other to reach the front of the queue at the teacher's desk. Mrs Winfield dishes out their marked-up "personal project" jotters[66], and then they scuttle back to their little plastic seats at their little desks to scan the grades within.

"Wait, wait! What did you get?"

A group of boys compare commentaries. Four of them have done their projects on 2002's FIFA World Cup. Some have fared better in the final marking than others.

I wait patiently to retrieve my pièce de résistance, '*Golf: A Beginners' Guide*'. Hours had been spent on this opus, fastidiously researching golfing lingo (this was pre-internet, so most intel was from my dad's golfing books and...interviewing my dad) and drawing less-than-flattering

[66] Scottish slang for 'exercise book'.

portraits of Tiger Woods and Colin Montgomery. Retreating back to my table to pore over the comments in peace, I flip to the marking sheet stapled onto the final page (after my glossary, acknowledgements, Ryder Cup-themed crossword, and refences section).

There lay the holy grail of primary five praise: a '*Mrs Winfield says 'Excellent Work!''* stamp *and* a gold star sticker. I read her comments, the serotonin train in my mind coasting to stratospheric new heights with each positive adjective written in green biro pen.

"What did you get, Kirsty?" One of the FIFA boys peers over my shoulder. "Holy cow! She got *fifty* house points!"

"What house are you in again?" another asks me.

"Kilravock," I reply. My cheeks are morphing into fireballs with embarrassment, but there's another emotion in the mix. I'm quietly chuffed that my hard work had paid dividends for others, too.

"*Yuuuus.*" He punches the air with a clenched fist in triumph. "We are so gonna win this year's House Cup."

Mrs Winfield later told the class how my personal project had helped her understand the golf match on the telly whilst she did her weekend ironing. Despite cringing at being the centre of attention, I adored the praise. I took the project home and showed my parents, who were equally effusive in their compliments. And so it began: that little book about golf was the gateway to becoming hooked on a lifelong quest to do well at everything I turned my hand to. Why? Did I long for external validation from others even at that age? I reckon it's more likely that trying too hard is encoded in my DNA.

Being type-A straight from the womb[67], my default setting was to thrive on achieving. And achieve I did. As my father likes to humblebrag within a vomit-inducing nanosecond of introducing me to anyone, I was awarded Dux (a prize given to the 'top' student) of both my primary and secondary schools. I was the student who got 99% in her Higher Physics exam, before garnering a slimline battery (AAA) in my Advanced Highers[68] and winning a scholarship to Oregon University (which I turned down at the thought of homesickness). Rather than leaning into teenaged rebellion, I was the friend who would be namedropped to parents as proof that a night out was definitely not going to be rowdy.

"You're the sensible one, Kirsty! Keep an eye on them, ok?" mums would half-jokingly, half-pleadingly tell me through rolled-down car windows after dropping off their daughters, as though I was a modern-day Florence Nightingale armed with a Samsung Razr lamplight on dingy disco dancefloors. It wasn't too far off the truth; conformist to the core, I was so goody-two-shoes that those two shoes would be bought from Clarks, with adequate arch support, cushioned soles, and a packet of blister plasters in my pocket for emergencies.

The more I succeeded, the more I *needed* to succeed, because I had a reputation to upkeep. There was a precedent set by always being in the top classes, but that veneer of easy perfection belied months spent revising. People would tell me not to stress about exams – "You, of all people, are bound to do well!" – blissfully unaware that their sentiment merely

---

[67] Born early on a Monday evening, I was in good time for my Mum to watch Coronation Street and ready to crack on with the rest of the working week.
[68] In chemistry, physics and maths, no less, because who wants an easy ride in their final year even when a university place is already guaranteed and there is literally nothing to be gained from getting good grades?

added to the pressure I felt to maintain my 'brand'.

Whilst my parents would frogmarch me downstairs on Saturday nights to watch Strictly Come Dancing rather than memorise the laws of thermodynamics, I did a great job at applying more than enough pressure on myself. Failure simply wasn't an option. Even worse, I only became satisfied when I achieved *more* than my own high-bar target. It's a toxic trait, for sure, but elements of this still remain in my personality today. Checking off excessive to-do lists, going above and beyond, still hits that sweet spot…if only temporarily.

Therein lies the crux: any pleasure derived from attaining my goals is always fleeting. I never fully enjoy accomplishments in fear of becoming complacent, or in case someone notices a flaw in my work, or that the banana peel of the universe will suddenly appear underneath my feet and I'll be exposed as an imposter. Pride comes before a fall, etc. There is a small part of me that feels that any goal is almost immediately devalued simply by my attainment of it; if *I've* managed to do it, it can't have been all that hard in the first place.

This thankless pursuit becomes even more poisonous when illness gets added to the broth, because chronic health conditions are not conducive to peak performance. They have a vampire-like ability to drain your focus, your drive, and your motivation, leaving you in the emotional and physical doldrums. For someone who wants to at least *try* to excel at almost everything, this realisation was (and continues to be) really bloody frustrating.

At the point of my liver disease diagnosis, I was operating my tried-and-tested pattern of {work hard + focus + goals + time + effort + discipline + being nice} = *success*. Yes, I'd loosened up a wee bit from school. But if I wanted to achieve a goal, then I would study how other people had done it, and then work like a crazed banshee to achieve it. I figured that a lot of the time, success boiled down to being prepared to put more effort in than 99% of people, sacrificing weekends, nights out, and romances. I'd get the extra books from the library, and attend the extra-curricular tutorials. This was not necessarily a healthy nor sustainable balance, of course, but such was the warped logic of my teenaged mind.

Illness detonated a series of explosions in this neat framework. No longer did I have a comfy physical buffer zone, a candle wick to burn at both ends, like other bright young things at university. There have since been many instances over the years where I've not be able to pursue an opportunity because something has flared or I've just felt crap (I cannot work more than eight hours a day, because my body tends to kickback with some nasty physical manifestation).

Diagnosis was the turning point that forced me to go easier on myself. My body unveiling itself as a fairground of dysfunction provided permission to stop pushing myself to reach that unobtainable state of 'perfection'.[69] The more I put myself in positions where I didn't have to be holistically type-A, the more I realised that being good enough was, well, *good enough.*

It's one thing being content with 'good enough' when we're talking about hobbies or work projects. It becomes a little

[69] Arguably my quest for perfectionism has merely leaked into other avenues, rather than being abandoned. Whilst liver disease has given me a free pass on certain self-expectations, it's also another opportunity to achieve. I try to 'excel' at being a patient; I'm the one who always tries to keep upbeat as though it's on me to keep NHS morale afloat with my jokes. I chase up on results very politely. The weirdest bit is I genuinely enjoy doing this.

trickier to navigate, though, when we're dealing with the big guns: the milestones I once expected to experience throughout my life. Truth is, I have often felt like an abject failure, both in terms of having a healthy body (my heart still sinks a little when seeing all the red-text results on my bloods report) but moreover in terms of checking off society's to-do list.

As much as we like to think we live in a liberal society where anything goes, and anyone can live their life as they wish so long as it doesn't cause anyone else any harm, we still put a lot of pressure on each other – and especially women – to follow the well-trodden path of marriage, homeownership, children and a pension pot. Which makes sense, I suppose, from a biological-procreation-of-the-species standpoint.

Nonetheless, it takes a lot – I repeat, *a lot* – of guts to turn your back (willingly or otherwise) on that path. When I was mid-20s, I still held onto a vague notion that, by 30, I would have at least some of the aforementioned deliverables under my belt. At 30, I sat down with a box of Maltesers for emotional support and reviewed the list. The only tick was against the pension pot. Even then, thanks to my liver function, I figured I probably wouldn't ever be old enough to reap the rewards of my Aviva 'mindful risk' portfolio.

I catapulted a handful of half-melted Maltesers into my cheeks and faced up to what I had been half-denying until that point: that my lifepath was different to that of my peers'. Graduation was my last communal life milestone check-in, and each year since then, I have felt a bit like Harry Potter[70] in the scene when he ventures into the maze at the Triwizard tournament – moving into the darkness, alone, unsure of the

---

[70] I'm aware I've referenced HP a lot in this book, however I'm not one of those millennials who is Potter-mad.

next turn, and getting further and further away from the cheers of the crowds.

I did a good job at kidding myself on in my early to mid-20s that my life wasn't *that* different, perhaps because most people's 20s are typified by a lack of concrete plans. Growing older, it became increasingly difficult to keep up with 'everyone else' without also feeling abnormal.

There was very much an element of resentment. It felt like everyone else was only now catching up with me in terms of maturity, after having their youth to be reckless, make mistakes and play fast and loose with life decisions. I've always felt I needed to get things right first time, be super sensible, or else face much more serious consequences. Sure, technically nobody was physically stopping me from doing lines of cocaine on a five-day bender in Ibiza, but I wasn't *stupid* (and to be fair, I probably wouldn't even enjoy this).

Playing the role of good girl every single day, despite not straying too far from my natural personality, is relentless. Add in having to put up with a degree of ridicule over the years from a small number of eegits for being 'too sensible', and it's easy to see why I was pissed off at feeling like I'd been left behind. In my 30s, it felt like I was starting to miss out on rites of passage that others were being afforded despite transgressions earlier in their lives. Everyone deserves a second chance and all that, but some of us don't have the privilege of screwing up the first one.

Accepting that life doesn't owe you any of the things that you once imagined it would is a bitter pill to swallow. It's made even harder when what life *does* serve up is a rather shitty alternative. But whilst the grief associated with accepting I won't – and in some cases, physically cannot – achieve what I might at one time have expected to, I can't assume that my life, had illness not been a part of it, would be any better or worse than the one I'm living now. Similarly, comparing myself to others' achievements will never change my situation. They're on their life path, I'm on mine. Neither of us will know the full backstory to each other's highlights reel.

Nonetheless, for someone keenly averse to risk, it's terrifying to suddenly realise that the tried-and-tested life map you've subconsciously been using as a reference point is now written in Latin and effectively unusable. I needed to be my own role model, when what I really wanted was for there to be a lifestyle equivalent of the coloured lines on the floor of my local hospital to guide patients to the right departments. For the first time, I had to really ask myself what I wanted to do with the life I had in front of me. In some ways, having to put restrictions on my plans made them fall into focus more sharply. A change in perspective, however daunting and forced it may feel, is an opportunity for improvement, or for doing things a little differently. And, actually, that has been liberating.

It helps to be a little bit stubborn. I recall accompanying my mum to a parents' evening during my second year of high school. We shifted round classrooms, sitting down at tables opposite each of my teachers, generally being told how well I was doing. So far, so boringly predictable. Then my final interview of the night – maths – threw a curveball. The teacher traced a bony finger along a laminated document with everyone's grades on the desk in front of her.

"Ah, yes. Kirsty." A thin smile stretched its way across her face. She was going to talk about my full marks in the previous week's unit test, surely. "Kirsty is well on her way to being selected for the Intermediate Two fast-track class next year."

I turned to mum and glowed with happiness. The night was a wrap. Back home for celebratory fish and chips, and –

"Well…" My teacher cut in to my reverie, her smile morphing now into a smirk. "…that is, unless *boys* get in the way."

My stomach churned with unease. Two universes which were still very far apart at that moment in time (my sexuality and my schoolwork) were in perilous danger of falling into each other's orbits. My face faltered for a bit, before I recomposed and smiled breezily.

"That won't distract me," I confirmed. This was all very embarrassing. Whilst walking home with Mum, I thought about just how determined I was to prove that teacher wrong. It's with that same level of stubbornness that I am determined to not let my illnesses stop me living my life, as far as I am able to.

Of course, there are moments when I get so frustrated by the impact of my illness that I question why I bother trying to do things differently. Or I'll second-guess my approach and wonder if it's all just an elaborate defence mechanism. Do I tell myself that my dreams weren't all they're cracked up to be, just to defend myself from the crushing realisation that they actually *were*, and I'm just never going to be able to achieve them?

Either way, if having a real sense of my own mortality has taught me anything, it's to stop wasting too much time thinking about whether to go for an opportunity. I tend to do a quick evaluation and then just go for it. Yes, I might not meet conventional checkpoints, but I'm determined to have as much fun as possible trying to work out which new ones I *can* reach instead.

There are practical limits, of course. It's all well and good when people say that a serious health scare gave them the motivation to 'follow their dreams'. The uncle-of-a-colleague you hear about through the grapevine who recovered from testicular cancer, then packed in his job as an accountant, started a podcast and is touring Thailand in a VW Camper. Conveniently, what people neglect to mention is that these wanderlust-ers often have lots of money to fall back on if it all goes belly up. For the rest of us, the live-for-the-moment mentality is not a viable option, because we still have bills to pay.

Society also likes to peddle the idea that everything is possible, if you want it enough. From early on in primary school, we're bombarded with some big questions wrapped up in innocuous guises – what do we want to do when we grow up? Aim for the stars, kids! But maybe, just maybe, we shouldn't teach our children that anything is possible if they want it enough and work hard, because that's simply not true. There are so many factors that can put obstacles in the way and divert plans off-course. I'm not saying we should suck the ambition out of their little souls, but instead, maybe to focus more on how to approach life with resilience.

And whilst we're at it, maybe lay off on the gold stars for the kids, too. Prepare them for an adult life that doesn't always come with ready-made awards for doing well. Yes, we have established means of cognisant societal approval when succeeding in ticking off certain milestones, but it's a shame we don't dish out recognition of the skills needed for navigating life's difficulties. Well done for getting through the emotional hurricane of your divorce; here's an 'excellent stamp' for how you managed your redundancy;

congratulations on paying for your mortgage single-handedly.

Like a Pavlovian reflex, my brain still expects praise from someone, somewhere, whenever I get a medical procedure, or take a new drug, or even when I do well in other areas of my life, like get a promotion at work. Because I don't normally make a big song and dance about my health (unbelievable, I know, given I'm writing a book about it), people don't understand (and how could they?) the extra hurdles I overcome to do anything in the first place. *Look at me!,* my inner child pipes up from time to time. *Am I not doing really, really well, all things considered? Praise me please!* It's about time I learn to be satisfied with a 'well done' from myself.

The reward for keeping on top of my appointments and attending clinics and getting bloods and chasing up on results and eating well and not drinking alcohol and taking medicines that make me want to throw up, is that I get to keep on living. No amount of external validation is going to provide a true understanding of the value of my health. Getting older, I like to think I care increasingly *less* about what others think of me anyways (and, newsflash, nobody really thinks of me at all, because we're all too wrapped up in ourselves).

Maybe my modern-day equivalent of Mrs Winfield's gold star lies in the appreciation I now have for the weeks in between blood tests when things are stable, or when I'm not in hospital, and not in pain, and not on a liver transplant waiting list. It's in the understanding that I don't necessarily need to be achieving expectations, or being productive. It's in knowing that sometimes, indeed often, the best moments are the ones I never expected, and that the perfection of my life lies precisely in its many, messy imperfections.

# ON CAREERS

"So tell us, Kirsty..." one of the three interviewers asked, exchanging a self-congratulating smirk with the others, "...why does one switch from studying chemistry to yearning for a career in asset management?"

*That, William-but-call-me-Will, is a very good question,* I thought. There had been an implicit expectation – from who, I'm not quite sure – ever since I was crowned Dux of my primary school, that I would go on to get excellent grades, and go to an excellent university, and get an excellent job, and generally 'do well'. Studying chemistry was a way to officially confirm to myself that I wasn't thick. I also fancied my Advanced Higher Chemistry teacher, which influenced my course choice, but I couldn't very well admit that to Will. To go back to his question: did I really want to work in a corporate ivory tower? No.

Rather than telling the truth, I fumbled out a response along the lines of how financial derivatives were the cornerstone of our society, securing the country's future in terms of pensions *yada yada*. This seemed to go down well with the panel. I took a sip of water from the glass emblazoned with the company logo. The man on the furthest left lifted his head and smiled.

"And finally, the clichéd HR question: where do you see yourself in five years' time?"

I fidgeted with the seam of my faux silk shirt which I'd bought in the Next Boxing Day sales. Despite it not yet bringing me much luck in the way of successful interviews, it was my best investment of 2014 because it required no ironing and matched with everything in my compact work wardrobe. The trio stared at me from the other side of the interviewing table, pens poised above notepads.

"Well, in five years' time, I want to…" I began with just the right amount of deliberation, honed through practise over the last two months of graduate scheme interrogations. This was the last question. *Don't,* I reminded myself, *for God's sake, say 'stay alive', ok? That's too on-the-nose, even if it's true.* Did I need to weave my chronic conditions into the answer? Legally, they were not allowed to let that sway their decision, but how could it not? And if I didn't tell them now, then when would I mention it? Better to just not bring it up. "…progress. I would like to see myself as having gained valuable work experience in different areas of the business, with a view to being considered for management roles in the years thereafter."

This generous serving of word salad, straight out of the *'Dummy's Guide to Corporate Bullshit',* prompted gentle nods on the other side of the table. I was singing sweet symphonies to their return-on-investment-hungry ears. Somehow, I had mastered the art of regaling clichéd responses with genuine feeling.

Like many fresh graduates, I plunged headfirst into a world of rejection, temporary internships and low wages. No employers seemed to care about my degree; knowing the difference between a tertiary amine and its stereoisomer was as useful in the real world as calculating the square root of a potato. Instead, employers wanted me to demonstrate my Outlook prowess.

The problem was, I had spent the majority of my final university summer holiday – the three months when anyone who's ahead of the game ensures they do a placement to get work experience – swirling round the revolving door of my local GP surgery, having bloods taken every Wednesday and crying over my hair falling out. Harping on about my ability to accurately measure a screaming baby's feet during my high school stint in Clarks was not quite going to cut it.[71]

Miraculously, I succeeded in my asset management interview, and commenced working at the company, despite, even to this day, being unable to fully explain what a financial derivative is. The whole experience was less 'Wolf of Wall Street' and more 'Little Red Riding Hood of Lothian Road', but I was just glad to have secured employment in Scotland.

Whilst some of my university friends were taking a more chilled approach – travelling, or taking time out to really think about what they wanted to do – I felt that I had no time to waste. I needed to get cracking with a career whilst I was still healthy enough, and I needed to stay in Scotland because that's where all my doctors were based, and where my familial support system was. Besides, travelling abroad was pretty much a no-no given the cost of travel insurance.

---

[71] Which is a shame, because fitting baby shoes is ridiculously tough.

Right enough, within months of starting that first proper job, I was faced with a particularly nasty flare of my AIH. This was when I learned that it's very difficult to maintain a glossy sheen of professionalism whilst my health turns into a burning dumpster truck.

Not wanting to take time off work, because I wanted to make the best impression, I would use the entirety of my lunch break to speedwalk across Edinburgh for blood appointments at my GP clinic (chucking a banana sandwich down my throat en route). I'd then return to my desk and pray that my phone wouldn't ring with bad blood test news. I recall one instance having to retreat hastily from the open-plan office to have a conversation with my hepatologist in the privacy afforded by… a toilet cubicle. Knowing I had five rings before it went to voicemail, I powerwalked across two departments to avoid missing the call and therefore having the anxiety of not knowing why the consultant called until he decided to try again.

"We're going to have to ramp your steroids up further to 40 milligrams, I'm afraid to say," he said. "It's best not to pussy-foot around with the dosage."

"It's just that I really hate being on steroids. They make me feel like rubbish and I don't want to take them if I can help it." I omitted the bit about the lack of appetite, the not being able to fit into any of my work trousers due to bloating, the rounded cheeks that made me look like a long-lost cousin of Alvin the chipmunk, the hair loss, mood swings and the general sense of impending doom that the higher-than-normal steroid dose I was already on had brought along to the party.

"Well, Kirsty, I've seen your liver numbers, and they are

indicative of very serious damage. If we don't stop this flare, then your liver will likely start to fail." He paused. "And I do not enjoy seeing my patients with failing livers. It is not nice."

I stared at the cubicle's floor tiles, my steroid-fuelled brain now producing a running side-commentary on the beauty of their little flecks of iridescent pearl which I'd never noticed before.

He continued. "Liver failure is precisely what we want to *avoid.* More steroids are the only way to go right now."

I bit my tongue to stop myself from crying. "Mmm."

Stepping out of the cubicle and into the bright lights around the fancy wall-length mirror, I could see that my purple eye bags were quite a spectacle to behold, contrasting vividly against what were now mildly-bloodshot eyes. I squeezed out some of the posh hand wash and slowly massaged my hands, rinsing them under the steaming hot water, sniffing away the little stream of cry-snot that had gathered in my nostril.

(If you ever need to pull an emergency stop on an emotional meltdown, I highly recommend a long look in a mirror, because there was something about seeing one's own blotchy, swollen face that immediately forces a deep intake of breath and brings about composure.)

I fired up the hand-dryer and, in an act of final resignation that I would indeed be ramping up on the steroids again, started dabbing the corners of my eyes to catch any wayward mascara. I pushed the big fancy door out into the big fancy corridor and walked back to my slightly less-fancy desk complete with ergonomic chair that did nothing to correct my terrible posture. I Ctrl-Alt-Deleted, popped in my password and reopened Excel to work out why Goldman Sachs were only registering a trade of three gold options at T+2, whereas we had reconciled 31. I became a corporate swan gliding across serene waters with her feet kicking like Michael Phelps underneath.

Work, and life, had to go on. There was a charade of normality to maintain. Rightly or wrongly, many of us have an inbuilt determination to 'do a good job' regardless of shitshows in our personal lives. To some extent, this mentality has been a coping strategy with which I level out the stress of my health conditions; professional work becomes a respite, or at least a distraction, from the other full-time job of keeping myself alive. It provides a sense of normality, of regularity, when everything else feels less secure.

For this reason, working is very important to me, and I consider it a privilege to be well enough to have a job. Flying in the face of all mental health mantras, I'll admit that work has always given me purpose and upped my self-esteem. I've inherited my parents' diligent work ethic and, whilst this may be alien to some people, I enjoy pushing myself. But – and it's a big but – the world of careers continues to be a personal minefield when it comes to managing my health.

Now, let it be said: I've been very fortunate to have relatively well-paid jobs which do not involve being out for 12 hours' physical labour each day. I'm not too stressed and have never worked excessive overtime. I can log in remotely if I'm totally fatigued, or want to avoid contracting office plagues which might then prompt another flare. I don't have to spend precious energy on commuting every day. My roles have provided a pension and additional sick leave benefits. Not everyone with chronic illness has these privileges.

But therein lies the rub: I've consciously made these 'safe' decisions, rather than following careers which may have played more into my interests…but would have been less accommodating health-wise. Having so many careers on offer, providing endless opportunities that no generation has had before, is hugely exciting. But sometimes I feel like I don't make the most of them, and it's incredibly frustrating to then feel too fearful because there's a little voice in my head saying that I shouldn't risk my health for the sake of a career boon. As much as I may *think* I don't let my liver disease influence my career ambitions, it absolutely does.

Billy Joel might say that Vienna will wait for me, and that I shouldn't worry because nobody is too old to switch paths. To some extent, I agree with him. I've been able to change roles across industries a few times. But what *he* doesn't realise is that it's a different kettle of fish when you're not quite sure if you're going to be fit for working in a year's time. Being on an invisible but very audibly ticking countdown to 'when, not if' a liver transplant is required carries with it a pressure to make sure any career choice is triple guaranteed by backup plans A, B and C. My margins for error feel tighter than everyone else's. If I need to retire early due to my health, I need to make sure I'm financially secure early, too. And that doesn't come easily.

Writing this down, it feels like I'm overthinking. I might not even live long enough for any of these worries to materialise. Equally, I need to be self-sufficient; I don't have generational wealth to fall back onto, and I'm not married, so financial security is a very real concern.

However, as I cruise into the wild west of my fourth decade, this cold pragmatism is confronted with a barrage of existential questioning. What do I really want my legacy to be, with the potentially limited amount of time I have on this planet? Is my work fulfilling?

Hardcore careerism is not in my bones. It possibly was, at one point, before I found out about the autoimmune problems. Whilst I like the *idea* of being a hotshot CEO, would scaling the corporate ladder lead me, a woman who is happy spending an evening on YouTube rewatching Strictly Come Dancing finals, to contentment? Unlikely.

The older I get, the more I'm happy to check out of the career-climbing competition, because it's not where my ambition lies (or at least, I'm pretty sure it isn't). Instead, I'll 'settle' for a job that affords me the time to find purpose outside of work.

Finding such a job is easier said than done, because there's more to a role than just the work itself. In my experience, a supportive manager is the determining factor between being able to pirouette successfully on the work-life-health tightrope, avoiding collapsing in a burnt-out heap in hospital.

If I'm having a flare of my illness, or if I've had a new diagnosis, my mind will – despite my best efforts – be prioritising my health a lot more than it will be focussed on my work. Some days, brain fog prevents me from being razor sharp during a presentation, and other times I'll need an afternoon off because I've had banding in the morning and am still as high as a kite from the sedation. Having a boss who understands that I'm not skiving, and instead encourages me to stay healthy, is the minimum that I expect in a workplace. Asserting this requirement of employers is a relatively new habit for me; before, I used to feel like I was being an inconvenience. Obviously, it's silly to feel this way, but being fresh out of university and operating in an ultra-competitive jobs market, I didn't want to be seen as the weaker link who wasn't pulling my weight.

It's worth noting that I felt this despite working in large corporate firms with modernised HR policies regarding disability and equal opportunity. In many workplaces, particularly in non-office-based roles or temporary work, there is still a gap in support available for people with chronic illness. On paper, businesses are legally obliged to 'make reasonable allowances' to help people with chronic illness or disability. In practice, some managers don't understand what this really entails, not necessarily through a lack of willingness to understand, but through an inability to grasp the holistic implications. Similar to how I can't imagine all the ways the birth of a child will impact a parent's life, it's inherently difficult for a person to understand the all-encompassing demands of a chronic illness on a life when they don't have a chronic illness themselves.

It's sometimes awkward having to forensically explain my condition to new colleagues. Why do I bother? Well, I feel I have a responsibility to. Firstly, I need them to understand why they should avoid me if they've got a cold, or why I nip out mysteriously during meetings (for bloods). Moreover, unveiling my own vulnerability usually helps to develop better relationships with people, which I hope makes me a more empathetic colleague. If anything, I probably overshare; my close colleagues know the high-level difference between colonoscopies, endoscopies and colposcopies, whether they wanted to or not. Yet, in doing this, I hope to reduce the stigma of both chronic illness and liver disease amongst people who might otherwise never be interested to learn about it.

The transplant conversation with bosses, however, never gets easier. I always cringe at my big reveal: "I might, one day, need a transplant…", ensuring to quickly follow it up with

"...but I keep really well right now, and that shouldn't happen anytime soon, and I take medications to keep me healthy".

Making my conditions sound less frightening or serious has become a habit. Again – why do I do this? Is it to make *other people* feel less awkward? Or is it because I feel obliged to downplay the risk of my condition becoming a blight on their resource plans?

The unpredictability of illness means that many roles are plainly unsuitable for those of us with chronic conditions, but there are also many cases where employers are stubbornly inflexible and don't make it easy for people to contribute as best they can. This makes me sad because, far from being a disadvantage, people with chronic illness often bring a perspective on life that is hugely valuable to the workplace.

Whilst many of us 'spoonies' have limited energy, we are usually pretty good at prioritising where to best spend the energy we *do have*. In fact, there are probably a lot of us who will go above and beyond the call of duty purely to prove – to ourselves or to society at large – that we are more than capable of holding down a job.

Being buffeted around by the unpredictable winds of chronic illness inevitably means we have been knocked down the steps of life a few times. Problems at work, when compared to the ones I deal with from a health perspective, always seem quite fixable. Since my stress-o-meter has seen peaks such as being told that one of my major organs is on the brink of failing, nothing at work ever feels *that bad*. Running a fruitless lessons learned workshop on design change is always preferable to getting an endoscopic procedure under sedation.

Granted, I'm not heading up a FTSE company. If I fail, the

shareholder price won't crash, and nobody dies. At any point in time, my life could be flipped around or cut short, and the rest of the world would move on without any disruption. With this in mind, I just try to do what I can, to the best of my ability.

At the end of the day, a job is a job. I'm replaceable in whichever workplace. But just as I could be swapped *out* of a role for someone else, so too could (with a stroke of bad luck), anybody who is currently healthy be swapped *in* for a life of chronic illness. People are not resources; they are real human beings, and there are far more important aspects to life than achieving career goals and making lots of money.

# ON WHAT I WISH I'D KNOWN AT 20

1. **Go easy on yourself.**

   Give yourself a break, kiddo. Learn to love yourself. You may want to extract your entrails and karate kick them into a different solar system from time to time, but take a deep breath, let that notion sweep past you like a rolling wave and bring it all back to a place of appreciation for your body keeping things somewhat together.

2. **Don't compare.**

   Social media is a plague on your mental health. It might be great for others, but you really need to wean yourself off Instagram. Tell LinkedIn to link off. Stop comparing your life progress to others', because you'll never win. Focus on pouring all your available main-character energy into making *your* life the best possible version. That said, be prepared to learn that this doesn't necessarily mean your life will exclusively feature things you *want* to happen.

3. **Self-advocate.**

   Attend all the appointments, get the blood tests, read the research papers, ask the questions, double check the facts, and keep banging your head off that bureaucratic brick wall, because it will eventually break. You won't get spoon-fed information on your illness, because ain't nobody got time to give you the full download.

   Be persistent. Don't listen to the GP who, upon telling them that you have pain every time you have sex, advises that they would "normally tell women to just have a glass of wine, but you can't do that, can you? So maybe just take a bath, and relax more". You're not (always) overthinking things. Your concerns are, more often than not, valid.

   Sometimes you'll be too bloody tired to think about doing all this, or too fed up, or just want a break from being a piggy in the middle who has to phone up hospital switchboards or trace unknown numbers or duel with a receptionist who makes the clinical decision that you're not 'vulnerable enough' to request bloods at home during the pandemic, even though your consultant has insisted you are, under no conditions, to go to the clinic. That's all totally valid, but unless you prioritise you, and keep on banging on the drum to get treated, nobody else will do it for you.

4. **Cry and shake your fists at the world from time to time.**

   Screaming into a pillow helps, but maybe go easy with that to avoid ending up with a face puffier than an inflated

Wotsit. Don't throw yourself too many pity parties though, ok, hun? Or, if you do, make sure they're not solo pity parties in your head, because they're the ones that tend to go on for the longest, and be the most self-destructive.

5. **Remember you're not a total freak of nature.**

Ever since you've been a teenager with no periods, you've felt a little bit like there's something a bit different about you. Something not quite right. Abnormal. Turns out, you were sort of right, but that doesn't mean you're a weirdo. So whenever you get treated like one, try to rise above it. Nobody is 'normal'. You deserve to enjoy your life just as much as everyone else.

And whilst we're on that, you'll soon learn that being diagnosed when you're younger will fast-track your ability to empathise. All of a sudden, you are now lumped in with the 'asterix' group; those 'severely immunocompromised with chemotherapy, HIV or long-term immunosuppression' who are called out specifically on medicine leaflets and advised to check everything with a doctor. You realise that, far from being outcast lepers in intensive care wards, these are people like you, out there, living their lives. This will teach you that serious illness can happen to anyone at any point in their life. This level of maturity will become one of your strongest assets, allowing you to connect on a deeper level with people.

6. **Exercise.**

No-one's asking you to cheerlead at an international CrossFit convention, but a notional effort to get a wee walk in a few times a day, and get the heart pumping a few times every week, really pays off physical and mental dividends.

Being fit-ish helps so much in terms of recovery from illness, mobility and joint problems.

7. **Take stock of what you do have.**

There's a perverse game you will end up inventing called 'It Could Be Worse' (and it's not in any means the right approach to take[72]) whereby, if something goes wrong or you get ill or an infection or whatever, you will try and imagine all the different ways that the situation could be worse.

For example, if you get a skin infection and the antibiotics used aren't okay to use with a poorly liver, you'll think – well, it could be worse, my car could also break down, and I could have Covid and then be sent to prison, falsely accused of murder. There's always another raft of problems that can be added to a list of problems, and this game gives you a moment's peace from the worry over the original problem by imagining all the different ways that it could be ten times worse. Win-win.

8. **Talk about how you feel, and listen to the response.**

Be vulnerable. Be honest. Whether it's moaning to your family, or chatting with friends, or working with a therapist, or writing it all out on a laptop, it's healthy to express

---

[72] I'm aware that this game is not going to be appearing as a coping mechanism on any psychological self-help books (if it does, then I'm trademarking it and you saw it here first), but it helps me to retain a morsel of perspective. I'm not downplaying the original problem or beating myself up for feeling down about it. It goes without saying that I'm the only person who's allowed to play '*It Could Be Worse*' with my problems.

yourself. Articulating worries helps to really drive to the heart of my problem, or sometimes just find that expressing yourself in a different way unlocks an alternative personal reflection or provides the opportunity to receive a solution you would otherwise not reach. It becomes unhealthy when you keep rehashing old ground and not getting any further forward with the processing bit – if this happens, then for the sake of your mental health and for your personal relationships it's probably best to see someone professional.

9. **Try to find something to smile about, and reflect that smile out to the world.**

Even if you feel like shit. Even if you're a little bit hopeless. Even if everything's gone tits up, try to make a joke of it. You'll find that this helps things become a little bit less scary. Your sense of humour is your saving grace. Never take yourself, or your situation, too seriously.

It takes a lot of strength to have bad stuff happen to you and not spit that back as anger or cynicism into the world. Seek to become the type of positive person that you wish there were more of in life. Try to keep making the world seem that little bit better for you being in it. You'll find that feeling is ultimately rewarding.

10. **Be a human Nike Swoosh and Just Do It.**

You don't have guaranteed time on Earth, and you know it. Stop procrastinating and doubting yourself, and just do the thing. If you really, desperately want something, there's usually (not always, but usually) a way to do it or adapt it to some extent. And if you can't, then at least give it a damn good shot at exploring all your options so that you can say that at least you tried.

Apply for that creative writing course, try that laughter yoga session, travel round Europe on a train, go on dates. Within reason, don't let your health get too much in the way of squeezing as much juice from your life as you possibly can. It's clichéd, I know – but life is for living, and you take those nasty drugs every damn day to help you do just that. Make it worth it.

# ON ALCOHOL AND STIGMA

The stationary section in a genteel countryside café's gift shop isn't the first place that springs to mind when imagining situations necessitating content warnings, but the universe works in mysterious ways, and it was whilst browsing the selection of birthday cards that I became more triggered than Mary Whitehouse accidentally walking in on a swingers' soirée.

The threshold to get me on my high horse is admittedly low, but nonetheless I found myself overwhelmingly peeved to find that, amongst the four rows of cards on offer, no fewer than nine related to alcohol.

The first showed an innocuous faux-dictionary page.

*Alco-hole (NOUN): A gap in your memory left by an alcohol-induced blackout*

The card next to that showed a couple of twig-legged cartoon characters flopped over a sofa, emblazoned with the tagline:

*Who is this 'moderation' we're supposed to be drinking with?*

My blood pressure steadily rising, I eyed yet another one, this time with a goblet of red vino on the front.

*Wine: Because everyone needs a hobby*

Just before I forced myself to walk away, a Ladybird-Books-inspired design crept out from the back. A cartoon Blackbeard raised a bottle towards the viewer:

*Drinking rum before noon makes you a pirate, not an alcoholic!*

Maybe I'm too sensitive, and maybe I need to learn to take a joke at face value. But I'm also prepared to die alone on a hill with one bony finger pointing to the fact that what may be intended as small and inconsequential witticisms are, instead, symptoms of a worrying attitude towards alcohol that seems to pervade our society today in the UK.

Alcohol: the social lubricant that has the mysterious power to get parties going but also facilitate frictionless downward spirals more effectively than a deluxe version of WD40. I struggle to name another carcinogen which we glamorise the overconsumption of, whilst simultaneously vilifying those gripped by its addictiveness.

Putting aside wider societal attitudes momentarily, alcohol is a prickly topic even within the liver disease community itself. When I was first diagnosed, every patient information leaflet advised caution over the use of social media. Whilst Facebook might be helpful in providing a sense of community, the guidance noted, it might also prove to be a breeding ground for ill-informed comparison with other patients. In my experience, there are often two distinct camps defining the liver disease community:

1. Those whose liver condition is caused by alcohol misuse, and

2. Those for whom alcohol is not a part of the picture.

Despite good intentions, what this means in practice is that there's often a covert superiority flex primed to spring into action. For the most part, everyone gets along swimmingly, sharing common lived experiences and lending much-needed positive prayers ahead of blood tests or providing words of comfort over concerns of organ rejection. But it only takes one naive newcomer to ask, *"Do you drink alcohol after your liver transplant?"* for the Facebook equivalent of a barbed hand grenade to be detonated on an otherwise mundane Wednesday night.

Tribal allegiances emerge from the murky undergrowth, niceties are sidelined, and thinly-veiled judgement barges in. Janice says that she *"would never touch alcohol again, but then I never drank much before my diagnosis anyway, so it's not a problem for me"*. Bob counters this with a *"One drink doesn't hurt from time to time, surely! As long as drink wasn't the cause of your liver condition in the first place - life is for living, after all!"*. Lucy reacts with an unhappy face and rebuts with an explanation of why she *"would never risk my precious gift of a transplant by letting so much as a drop of alcohol slip through my lips"*.

It's easy to understand how an innocent question can spark a wildfire that burns away until a moderator rushes in with the fire-retardant foam to dampen the keyboard flames. Sometimes it's less overt damnation of alcoholism, but more of a subtle dig.

A new member of the Facebook group will, for example, introduce themselves via a diagnosis story, explaining how their GP assumed that their liver damage was caused by drinking too much alcohol. They'll explain how horrified they were to even be considered in this way, given that the most they drank was a glass of wine once a week.[73] "And I've never done drugs or *anything like that,*" they'll add with an online voice dripping with prejudice, as though alcoholism wouldn't happen to *someone like them.*

Thing is, I'm guilty as charged. Whenever I explain my liver disease – be it to nurses, colleagues, the friendly woman I sat next to on a flight to Amsterdam – I feel compelled to dispel any doubt around my condition being inflicted through misuse of drink or drugs. I've never been on the receiving end of stigma from a healthcare professional, but many liver patients have. Indeed, studies have shown that a whopping 73% of patients with liver disease have reported being a victim of stigma, and 29% have reported that such stigma has stopped them from accessing appropriate medical care.[lxix]

Why do I feel the need to distance myself from any association with alcoholic liver damage? Do I believe that, if my cirrhosis was *not* autoimmune, I would be any less deserving of sympathy? Do I worry that I'd be judged? And if that *is* the reason, why should alcoholism be considered differently to any other condition?

The answer, I fear, lies somewhere between social

---

[73] I do sometimes wonder if liver disease has a habit of selecting people who never drink.

conditioning and misinformation. There exists a dichotomy in the way our society addresses alcohol. It is a drug which we worship and fear in near equal measure, depending on the context. Middle-class binge drinking – *good*; working class alcoholism – *bad*. We steer clear of the man sleeping on a park bench nursing an empty bottle of Tesco Value gin, we litter conversations with disdainful descriptions of local 'alkies' or 'druggies' or 'drouths', we keep our eyes diverted, our sniggers suppressed, when we swerve past the tracksuit-clad woman swaying along the pavement with her bottle of Buckfast belting out an out-of-tune song at ten in the morning.

Yet yummy mummies will happily sign up to boozy bottomless brunches and stock up on those cards in countryside shops with just-joking-but-not-really taglines glamorising what is, in any other context, misuse of alcohol. Nobody would ever think of buying a card with a cheeky pun about how shooting up heroin makes you a rock star, not a drug addict. When I told my university director of studies that I had liver cirrhosis due to an autoimmune liver disease, he scribbled down some notes to apply for extenuating circumstances, and (presumably trying to lighten the mood) added with a half-chuckle: "God, well, I'd hate to see the state of *my* liver these days."

Who decided where we draw the line? Nobody bats an eyelid when you say you don't smoke. If you admit you're vegetarian, people won't look for evidence of a previous life. Yet it's intriguing how many people query why I'm avoiding a known group 1 carcinogen[74] and settling on the lemonades, instead. Explaining that liver disease is the reason why I don't

[74] These are considered to be chemicals with sufficient data to indicate they cause cancer in people. Other carcinogens of this type include asbestos and acetyl aldehyde.

drink[75] is usually sufficient to silence those who ask, but sometimes saying "end-stage liver damage" just doesn't quite penetrate their dense cerebrum, and people want to dig deeper. It's tricky to decide what is more impolite: to graphically describe cirrhosis, or to tell them to piss off.

There have been occasions when people feel that their degree in gastroenterology from the University of Knows-fuck-all qualifies them to assure me that having a G&T won't affect my liver. Take Seamus (not his real name) who tagged along with my group on a night out. Having overheard my order at the bar, he decided to launch into a modern-day Spanish inquisition.

"Coke?" His face screwed up as he motioned towards my high-ball glass. "That's no kind of proper drink."

I swirled the lonely lime segment (this was a posher Wetherspoons) around with a straw. "It's fine."

"Why aren't ya drinking?"

"I don't drink."

"Oh, aye? Why not?"

I glared at him, almost impressed that even with Dutch courage, he had the balls to ask this. "I've got a liver problem," I shouted, competing with Pitbull's dulcet tones being blasted out from the speakers.

"Oh." Little cogs churned behind his eyes as he processed

[75] Whilst one alcoholic drink probably won't do that much harm, it probably won't do much good, either. I just avoid drinking altogether because I don't even like the taste of alcohol and it's just not worth it.

this information. I hoped this would stop his questions. Alas, Seamus enjoyed playing the role of D.I. Dickhead a little bit too much.

"But, I mean, *one* drink isn't going to kill you, is it?"

I sucked up a paltry gulp of Coke-infused water to cool what was now an internal rage burning up from his audacity. I spun round slowly on the bar stool and stared square into his slightly off-focus eyes.

"Mind your own fucking business, Seamus."

I didn't say that, of course, because, at 23, I was still far too insecure, polite and confrontation-averse to say what I should have. Instead, what I *actually* said in response was:

"Well, no. I won't take a sip of vodka and, like, keel over dead." My voice at this point broke slightly and my blood pressure was so high that my inside wrist was visibly vibrating. "But I don't have a good liver, so I don't drink, okay?"

He put his hands up in mock defeat. "Okay, okay. Whatever. *Fine.*"

Another time, I refused the offer of a small glass of Bucks Fizz at a boyfriend's parents' house, only for his mum to double check: "I know you don't drink, but there's hardly any alcohol in a Bucks Fizz, is there?" Not wanting to make a fuss or have to explain why I shouldn't, I accepted her offer and nursed an untouched flute for the rest of the evening.

For my birthday, a different boyfriend gifted me a bottle of prosecco as we sat down to a family dinner. Maybe I hadn't been clear enough by not drinking in all the time I had known him, or in all our deep chats where I laid bare my fears about losing my hair as a direct result of the steroids I was taking to stop my liver inflammation.

"Thanks," I pulled a smile from the depths of my people-pleasing reserve as I lifted the bottle out from the carrier bag. *Don't look disappointed. Don't get upset. He's travelled for five hours to spend your birthday with you. Don't show him you're beyond offended at what is possibly the worst present he could ever have chosen.*

"That's for when you get well again," he shuffled around in his seat, shifting out the way of the jet-stream of poisoned darts fired from my sister's eyes over the dinner table.

"But I won't ever get…" I sucked my lips under my teeth to stop them quivering. "Cool. Thanks."

When I was diagnosed, I found one of the most difficult challenges was having to explain my diagnosis to each of my friends, and tell them the reason why I couldn't drink anymore. I tried to keep it upbeat: *oh, it's no big deal. I'll be fine. You'd never know to look at me, right? Cokes are on you, though – ha!* Deep down, though, I was really scared. Not of being unable to drink, but of losing that connection to my peers. Most university social events came hand-in-hand with a vodka, lime and lemonade.

For most of my 20s, I spent too much time apologising for not drinking, for being too quiet or too boring, or for leaving parties[76] early. Coupled with this self-inflicted guilt complex, I spent a lot of time being toxically resentful of others my age who could and would drink – and drink, and drink – whilst being blissfully unaware of liver enzyme levels or bilirubin

[76] The truth was, most of the parties were boring because everyone got pissed, and there's nothing less scintillating than a sober conversation with a gibberish drunk.

thresholds. On a chemistry student group night out, I watched with a mixture of pity and fury as a young lad started – and simultaneously ended – his evening by vomiting pure bile on the street at 11pm. It was a classic, if extreme, tale of someone who didn't know how to handle his drink, and I recall two paramedics bundling him into an ambulance. Rumour in the lecture theatre the next day was that he had to be treated for alcohol poisoning.

Watching people line up woozily at nightclub bars to buy their ninth tequila shot, I'd have an urge to run over and shake their shoulders. *You're so lucky to have a working liver, don't fuck it up. Take it from me, you don't want to deal with a failing liver. I don't want to be fighting you in the queue for a liver transplant in ten years' time. Look after your body.*

Such thoughts tend to ruin the fun, so I found myself not going on nights out. It took years to learn how to get over that envy and to work through those destructive thoughts. To stop wasting my energy judging how others are living their lives, and instead start focussing on how best to live my own.

I still get indignant. I still look at some people with disdain when they're falling over drunk, or when others gloat about how "fucked up" they're going to get on a night out. I've just learned how to better counter these thoughts with the understanding that nobody is perfect.[77]

More positively, it feels like sobriety is trendier now than it was when I was younger. Gen Z seem to be more accepting of individual choices and overall healthier lifestyles, with binge drinking not holding the same appeal amongst youngsters as it

---

[77] Although Ryan Gosling comes very close. God help me, Ryan, if you ever become problematic, then everything I think I know and understand about the world will crumble to dust.

did back in the early 2010s.

Nonetheless, it is still frustrating to see a lack of awareness of liver health amongst the wider population, despite it being estimated that liver disease will overtake cardiac problems as the number one leading cause of death in the UK over the next 30 years.[lxx] The liver can be damaged without obvious warning signs, and liver disease is a ticking timebomb which could explode en masse in the next few decades. We're sleepwalking right into it.

I believe that, as a society, we need to take a long, hard look in the mirror and confront our warped and hypocritical attitude towards alcohol. It's not popular, but we need to promote healthier lifestyles overall and encourage more responsible drinking. We need to address the deeply complex socioeconomic issues that contribute to addiction and alcohol misuse.

There is so much to be done. I'm not suggesting that all-out prohibition is the way to go – to be clear, I'm not advocating for any specific policy, because I'm nowhere near a qualified expert on the issue – but perhaps a good first step would be for us to be more mindful of all the small ways in which we validate unhealthy attitudes towards alcohol, and to stop buying those stupid cards in the giftshops.

# ON BABIES (OR LACK THEREOF)

While some girls spent their youth pushing those weird baby dolls (the ones that yelped when you squeezed their left foot) around playgrounds in elaborate prams, I was moonlighting as a theme park magnate on a PC game called Rollercoaster Tycoon. Whole evenings were spent building flume rides and working out how to profit from selling umbrellas when it started raining in my imaginary worlds.

One snowy afternoon in primary six, my entire class was forced to sit cross-legged on the floor whilst the big TV was rolled in front of us. What we thought might have been a pre-Christmas treat – Mrs. Doubtfire, or The Santa Clause – transpired to be a disturbing sex education video featuring a woman giving birth in all its unapologetic goriness.

Quite why Channel 4 felt this graphic bloodbath was a necessary addition to the otherwise entirely animated programme is anyone's guess, but it proved to be a highly effective contraceptive for the next nine years of my life. In between the heart palpitations I had whilst watching it, a distinct *whooshing* started in my ears. My body was overcome with that specific clamminess that precedes fainting, and my mouth ran dry. The mere thought of having to experience *that* kind of childbirth made me want to vomit. Years later, with a lack of periods as a teenager, I had an uneasy sense that nature didn't have me pinned down as a mother, either. Call it foreboding, if you will.

Fast forward to today, when social media's algorithm of doom decides to show me that one of the elaborate pram girls from school is now on her *fourth* real-life baby. I swipe through photos of the cherub, who is crowned with an elasticated headband and plonked down next to a printed card showing her age in gold-embossed cursive font.

Women who I last saw at university in 2013, halfway to hypothermia at three in the morning whilst queuing for a double portion of chips and cheese after a night spent dancing to Avicii's *Levels*, are now routinely popping up on my Instagram feed. They're all sporting perfectly rounded beach-ball bellies under White Stuff sundresses on 'babymoons' in Sardinia, or the Maldives, or somewhere equally as fancy.

My initial reaction is one of amazement, because in my head we're all still 21. How are they going to manage a baby *and* passing their exams? What about getting jobs? Then my lagging brain catches up and concludes that, no, it's just me who's living in a time warp. It's perfectly reasonable for these 30-something women to have had enough offspring to fill a hatchback car. Compared to just two generations ago, they're positively running *behind* schedule. And then it dawns on me that I need to start paying attention to the area which I've been deliberately avoiding thinking about for most of my 20s: whether I want to have children, or not.

When it feels like many women my age are falling pregnant faster than you can say *increased human chorionic gonadotrophin levels,* it's easy to underestimate how much of a Herculean effort is required to i) get pregnant, ii) stay pregnant, and iii) deliver that baby. Even if the mother is blessed with a clean bill of health, pregnancy is a huge physical strain on a woman's body.

Take, for example, blood during pregnancy. The total volume in the body increases by 20-30%[lxxi], depending on the stage of the pregnancy. This means the mum's heart must also grow bigger, to pump all this extra blood around, which can put extra pressure on the organ.

Ready for another bit of pregnancy trivia? Normally, the pancreas makes a hormone called insulin which helps control blood sugar (glucose) levels. During pregnancy, some women experience gestational diabetes, whereby the hormonal changes from pregnancy cause the body to not make enough insulin. Glucose then builds up in the blood, which can cause a raft of complications.[lxxii]

It's a wonder that any pregnancy goes to plan. Modern medicine is great and all, but there are limits. Pregnancy (and childbirth) is still inherently risky[78], and when things don't go smoothly, it is arguable that society isn't adept at talking openly about it.

Given these are the risks in a healthy mother, consider falling pregnant when your body is already struggling to toe the line of being well. If that line is, as it is for me, the

[78] Anyone who's read Adam Kay's brilliant 'This is Going to Hurt' will understand how badly things can go wrong in obstetrics.

difference between maintaining compensated liver function and falling into the dark chasm of potential liver failure, then the odds of a dangerous pregnancy are upped substantially.

First off, pregnancy puts added strain on almost all organs. Not only do the heart, kidneys, lungs and liver need to continue their day job of keeping mum alive, but they also need to support baby, too. The mother's needs are demoted to second place, and everything is pushed around to optimally accommodate baby. If, as is the case with my compensated cirrhosis, the potential mother's organs are only just about managing to keep *her* going from day to day, then a baby makes complex additional demands of organs that are running on empty.

With increased blood volume comes a raft of additional complications such as an increased likelihood of varices in the portal vein and therefore spontaneous (and potentially lethal) bleeding. A frequent variceal banding programme to keep a close eye on things would be par for the course in any cirrhotic-mother pregnancy, but each banding session could, in itself, pose risks to both mother and baby.

Then we have the meds. After the thalidomide catastrophe in the 20$^{th}$ century, an ever-increasing abundance of caution is used in the prescription of any drug during pregnancy. Some drugs simply cannot be taken for the sake of the baby's safety, and certain immunosuppressive drugs are absolute no-goes. This means that some ladies with autoimmune problems need to switch medication prior to conceiving, and risk inducing a flare or worsening of their disease.

And that's before we even consider the hurdle of any *additional* medication that might be required whilst pregnant. What if I had a flare during my pregnancy, and needed to take high-dose steroids? What impact would that have on a growing baby? Furthermore, as pregnancy is a period of natural dampened immune response – the body is itself trying hard to not attack the 'foreign object' growing inside – it is not unheard of for autoimmune activity to wane temporarily. But this means that the body's innate ability to counteract infection is also reduced.

This reduced immunity, along with long-term immunosuppression and cirrhosis, would create a further-increased susceptibility for infections. Hypothetically speaking, if I was pregnant and required antibiotics, then there is a good chance that a great number of treatment options would be ruled out due to i) the pregnancy itself ii) impaired liver function due to cirrhosis or iii) contraindications of some of my other regular medication. It's a bit of an all-round shitemare that could ultimately leave either the baby or me seriously ill.

The physical dangers of a pregnancy in my current state of health are clear. Not long after being diagnosed, I spent hours poring over research articles outlining how women with cirrhosis are more likely to miscarry, experience higher incidences of stillbirth, or end up with liver failure post-partum. There is very limited data on cirrhotic mothers, because whilst conceiving and giving birth with cirrhosis isn't unheard of, it is pretty rare.[lxxiii] Maybe, I thought, I was healthier than the ladies in these research papers. Maybe motherhood could still happen for me. I never pressed for answers from doctors because I was quite happy to live with that hope. Besides, I felt somewhat safe in the knowledge that any consideration of babies was strictly reserved for my 30s.

And until very recently, no doctor had ever sat me down and said directly, in a non-roundabout way, that it *wouldn't be possible* to have children with my liver being poorly.[79] I'd had it explained to me that I should definitely, *absolutely*, keep taking contraception because it 'wouldn't be a good idea to get pregnant'. I was told that there have certainly been healthy pregnancies in post-transplant patients. But nobody wanted to be the one to sit me down and say: *Look. You're just not going to have a child with your liver as it is right now.* And to some extent, I get it. Then, one day, not long after turning 30, I received a letter from a fertility clinic that categorically stated that it would be incredibly dangerous for me to become pregnant in my current state (I talk more about this in my IVF chapter).

Some doctors don't like dealing in hypothetical situations. They maybe didn't think the discussion was worth having until I rocked up with a partner-in-waiting, clinging on to a failed Clearblue stick. When I made a comment at a colposcopy[80] about potentially removing my cervix (which, at that point, didn't seem to be able to clear itself of HPV) if I was unable to have children due to my cirrhosis, the doctors made it clear that they wouldn't consider it because I was 'too young' and 'might change my mind about having children'.

But this time is now running out. I'm getting older. That 'biological clock' is ticking, but it's unhelpfully joined by its less famous cousin, the 'liver transplant' clock. Realistically, my only hope of falling pregnant would be with a new liver. And do I want to hasten my need for a transplant purely for the sake of being in with a chance of having biological children? Absolutely not.

---

[79] Though a rheumatologist did tell me at 20 (before my liver disease diagnosis) that if I wanted to have children, I would be best having them *then*, before my lupus got worse. I laughed in her face, because I had a grand total of £3.50 in my current account at the time and had never had a boyfriend.

[80] A procedure to examine the cervix with a microscope and some acids. I get one every six months to do a more thorough check on abnormalities detected in my smear tests.

Whilst I don't often wish I was a man, it's at times like these I think it might be a little simpler to not have ovaries. Dipping into my *'let's choose to completely forget about this'* memory box, I recall going out for a first date with someone who (in between moaning about his ex-girlfriend who, it transpired on the date, he still lived with) was the type of man to dive straight in with big life questions.

"So…" he cleared his throat whilst sweeping some crumbs off his knee, "…do you want kids, then?"

I choked on a limp chip. This question was somewhat left field, considering we were only just debating whether Netflix was worth the subscription fee. I paused to let my brain figure out if I even needed to answer this, and if I did, how best to frame my response. *Keep it light. Even when it's not light, at all, because this whole topic is incredibly raw and painful. But don't put a downer on the date. Just say, breezily, something along the lines of –*

"Well, I suppose I've never been in a relationship where children have been even remotely on the horizon, so I've never had to think too deeply into it."

It was hard to gauge what his reaction was, because he was too focussed on picking out tomatoes from his side salad. An awkward silence fell upon the table and I felt obliged to fill it with information that really was better left unsaid. *Don't say it, Kirsty, don't say it… oh, ok, you're saying it.*

"But I probably won't be able to have children. I've, er, got a liver condition. It makes it kind of difficult to get pregnant."

Narrowing his eyes, he took a long sip of his beer, before smacking his lips together with an exaggerated exhale.

"Lucky you." A snort of laughter – yes, ladies and gentlemen, *laughter* – escaped as he re-aligned his beer's coaster at right angles to the edge of the table. "I hate children. Wouldn't want to have them. In fact, you couldn't *pay me* to have them."

I scanned his face for a glimmer, even a fleeting hint, of empathy, regret or self-awareness, but as this wasn't forthcoming, I continued to stare at him in disbelief. He carried on with his rant.

"I've seen my sister's kids and they're absolute terrors. Expensive. Messy. Noisy. I don't know why anyone would actively choose to invite that chaos into their lives."

Unsurprisingly, there was no second date, but for weeks afterwards, his words replayed in a loop in my mind. The reality of biology is such that this man could retire with his military pension (which, he boasted, was "very comfy") in eight years' time and decide that, actually, he *would* like to have children after all. He might go on to have a football team of babies and be glad that he reneged on his vow to childlessness. Oh, what I'd give to have that level of flexibility, to have the luxury of flipflopping between options in huge life decisions. It's the not having choices available that is the most painful aspect. Problem is, I don't think a man like him will ever appreciate this.

Receiving the letter from the fertility clinic catapulted me into months of reflection, not because my sole aim in life had been to be a mother (it had never been), but instead because of how close I am to my parents and sister. To me, a solid family unit is more valuable than having lots of money or career success; some of my happiest memories as a child were just chilling with my family on a picnic. I suppose I had assumed that I would be able to recreate this warmth in my own life, with my own children. Finally facing up to the reality that this wouldn't happen was a bit of a life earthquake.

I began to wallow in negative and defeatist thought cycles. Malicious sentiments would enter my head, amidst a background hum of *why me*, which would ramp up in volume at the merest hint of inconvenience. Then, within a matter of months, four friends announced pregnancies.

With every signing of a congratulations card, I was stewing in a toxic mix of self-pity blended with self-hatred for feeling anything *other* than complete happiness for my friends. I knew they would be happy for me if the roles were reversed. I felt like one hell of a bitch, but the unfairness of it all seemed overwhelming. Some of my friends had never had a blood test until they were pregnant. For others, going for their ultrasound scans was the first experience of being in a hospital. Meanwhile, I was clocking in at around 36 radiology appointments to check for tumours in my liver.

Initially, I wondered if I was envious of their ability to become parents, but over the next few months, my mindset shifted. With therapy sessions and many hours spent reading childfree blogs and Elizabeth Day books, I slowly realised that – *duh* – what I was feeling wasn't necessarily jealousy directed at my friends, but rather unprocessed sadness and frustration at my own lack of control, or agency.

I began to drill into the root of my sadness a bit further. Was I gutted at the thought of not having a mini version of myself walking around in the world? Had I dreamt of being pregnant and woken up disappointed? No. Did I see friends' babies and feel a pang in my heart for my own? In all honesty, seeing how exhausting parenthood could be made me *not* want to have children. Perhaps, then, having a child was more a 'thing to tick off the life list' in my head. I questioned whether my sadness was, in fact, not due to an inability to have biological children, but rather a form of grief for a version of my life untainted by the effects of a health condition.

Thinking about surrogacy, adoption, or being a stepmother to children of a partner doesn't fill me with warm, fuzzy feelings, and I wouldn't want to raise a child on my own. Whilst it's very difficult to understand how I feel about these alternative versions of motherhood when I'm not currently in a position to seriously consider them, there's a niggling sentiment at the back of my mind that grows stronger every day since being told it would be risky to do it biologically: do I *want* children in my life?

If, by some miracle, I was to get pregnant – say I had a transplant next year and it went swimmingly, and I also met the love of my life and decided that we want kids – I wonder whether it would be fair on that baby to bring them into a world where I might not be alive long enough to see them into adulthood. And yes, I know that technically everyone is in this boat when having children; nobody can predict the future. There are ladies post-transplant who have successful pregnancies and go on to live for many decades very healthily, which is brilliant. But I'm unsure if I, personally, feel that risk is outweighed by the potential for the love that I know I could offer a child.

Many people enter the world of parenthood blissfully unaware of everything that could go wrong – and it's just as well they do, or else nobody would ever have children. What if, heaven forbid, my baby *wasn't* healthy, or had my conditions, but none of the treatments worked? What if that baby had additional care needs for life? It's brutal to admit, but I think I'm too selfish to take such a gamble when I've already got a lot on my plate.

For now, I can always put my health above all else. If I need a nap to get my energy levels up, I can. If I can't work because I'm ill, the only person inconvenienced by not having that income is me. All the choices in my life are made based entirely on the needs of the key decision maker: me. The reason I've been able to stay so well for so long is due to my ability to be unapologetically self-centred. A baby would demand my priorities be readjusted, and my needs would necessarily be second to theirs. My health would be below the importance of keeping my child alive, and I'm not convinced I have sufficient wiggle room to do this. I'm not sure if, physically and emotionally, I could be the mum I would want to be.

I see some friends with children and realise how exhausting, stressful, demanding, boring and expensive (sorry to sound so transactional, but it's especially true in today's economy) parenthood can be. It's not all JoJo Bébé Maman babygros and trips to Peppa Pig World; it's bloody hard work. Whilst children are undoubtedly rewarding in many ways, I'm beginning to think that, given my circumstances, *not* having children has potentially larger positives.

If I had children before being diagnosed, I'd probably feel differently, but to some extent being told it was too dangerous has given me the permission to feel less guilty about not being able to have children, and even about potentially not really *wanting* to have them, either. Of course, it's ridiculous I feel like I need a 'free pass' in the first place, but such is the implicit pressure on women my age.

Am I completely 'healed' from being told I'm not going to

have my own babies without a liver transplant? Nope. I still feel a pang of *something* – I'm not quite sure what – when people announce their pregnancies, or discuss their children at work, or ask if I've got any plans for babies (and yes, people still do ask these kind of questions). The bottom line is that it sucks having to reconfigure life vision boards, time and time again. It's even worse when it's due to something completely out of my control.

This sense of unsolvable frustration will, I think, continue to upset me to some degree for the rest of my days. I will no doubt always grieve the alternative life I might have led with children and without illness. Yet as difficult as it may be to accept in its entirety, I believe that, given my situation right now, a childfree future is the best option for me.

# ON IVF

When the milestone of turning 30 loomed on the horizon, my brain started churning through the following thought process:

1. I didn't have a partner.

2. I didn't have periods.

3. Reasons 1 and 2 alone meant that I wasn't going to get pregnant naturally any time soon.

4. I had a reasonable amount of savings.

5. I was undecided as to whether I wanted to have children.

6. If I had a liver transplant whilst still relatively young (i.e. before mid-40s), there was a possibility, however small, that my body could be healthy enough to become

pregnant.

7. It would therefore perhaps be worthwhile 'harvesting' my eggs whilst I still had enough of them, and they were of a relatively good quality.

I asked my hepatologist whether it would be possible to freeze my eggs. Nothing ventured, nothing gained.

"It's a sensible question to ask. I suppose that would be an avenue worth exploring, but you'd have to kick all that off with your GP, rather than me,[81]" they advised.

Months later, after asking my GP twice for a referral (I'm still not quite sure what happened to the first request), I found myself in the waiting room of a fertility clinic. Passing time before my initial appointment, I inspected the health posters adorning the walls.

One had a stream of white smoke emanating from the bellybutton of a ballooned pregnant abdomen, as though it was housing the next Pope. *"Every cigarette harms your baby. Support is available to help you quit."* Another showed a heavily pregnant woman sipping from a glass of wine, the rosy liquid winding its way down her throat and leaking out over an inexplicably neon blue foetus. *"When you drink, your baby drinks too. The safest choice is no alcohol at all during pregnancy."* I wondered if other women who had visited this clinic – women who would drain their pension funds in order to fall pregnant, women who have tried fruitless cycles of pumping themselves full of hormones, women who refrain from eating meat and

[81] As the world now offers a PhD in Taylor Swift songs, I reckon the world should also offer a PhD in NHS bureaucracy. This would cover the peculiar phenomenon whereby finding the crew of the Mary Celeste would be easier than trying to negotiate the system to get what you need.

religiously take folic acid and would do anything, *anything,* to fall pregnant – see these posters too, and feel a similar sense of despondency. Of unfairness. Of trying so hard to do everything right but still being taunted by reminders that there are people out there who have the privilege of doing everything wrong. So many people, in fact, that the NHS need to have public health posters to advise against these behaviours.

I chose to survey the waiting room instead. A couple who, based on their fresh-facedness, I surmised to be in their late 20s, planted themselves – the lady a little more slowly, being around seven months' pregnant – on the seats opposite. The man started mindlessly scrolling through his phone. He showed her a funny video; she rolled her eyes before beginning to flick through a wad of information leaflets. I imagined how they will fare in a few months' time. Will they have a wee boy? Will the delivery be straight forward? Will he help with night feeds? Will she go back to work? Will they have one more?

One of the cruellest aspects of infertility lies in those moments when you're forced to sit amongst the most overtly fertile women, waddling around with their swollen bellies and hormonal glow, in hospital waiting rooms. No matter how often I'm lumped in amongst mums-to-be, it never gets any *easier.* It's not even restricted to fertility clinics; the same thing happens in other clinics too, like the colposcopy and gynaecology clinics I attend.

I'm not suggesting that there should be a ban on pregnant women being in at the same time as me – the world doesn't stop moving just because *my* body doesn't work – but every time it happens, it's like a searing third-degree burn to my ovaries. I look at these women, sometimes with their partners, or sometimes accompanied by their own mothers, and I can't help but project blissfully happy futures for them all. I see them taking the baby home from the hospital, I see the baby's first steps and first teeth and bedtime stories, and nursery pickups and school runs and holidays and graduation ceremonies. I see them having a future that I once thought might happen for me, too.

It's delusional, I know. The life I create for them is a saccharine-sweet, idealistic version of motherhood. I'm not including the traumatic births and perineal tears, sleep deprivation and mastitis, or temper tantrums and perpetual parental anxiety over the future of that child. But that doesn't stop me from doing it.

Anyway – back to the fertility clinic. A nurse called me through for a urine sample. But wiping myself after, I noticed a pinkish hue on the loo roll. In what can only be attributed to the universe confirming that my life is a big practical joke, I appeared to be having the faint traces of…a period. Despite having nothing – no spotting, *nothing* – in the three years since having my IUD inserted, my weird and wonderful body had decided to start bleeding minutes before I was going to get an internal ultrasound. Wonderful. After explaining the situation – *I'm sorry, I never normally have a period, I'm not quite sure what my body is playing at, please don't think I'm a total eejit* – I was assured by the nurse that, unless I was flowing like the River Ganges, it should be okay to proceed.

I wish I could say that was the lowlight of the appointment. Alas, it was not. I was called through to the consultant, whose opening gambit, a dagger straight to my heart, was:

"So, Kirsty, you're here today because you're on the transplant list, and your partner and you would like to explore the options of egg freezing, right?"

To this day, I'm unsure how the lines of communication between my GP referral and the clinic got so profoundly crossed, but nevertheless I took a yoga-esque deep breath and explained that, *no*, I was very much single, and *no*, I was very much still running off a cirrhotic liver, but *yes*, I wanted to find out if I could freeze my eggs.

"Oh. I see. Sorry about that confusion." She backspaced an entire text box on the PC screen. Not for the first time in my NHS patient career, I just smiled and nodded.

We ran through the health checklist: no smoking, no drinking, no illegal drugs, no family history of infertility, nor any other health problems. Normal BMI. Good diet. Abnormal smears since my very first test, which were being followed up twice a year with colposcopy and cervical biopsy. No regular periods except for when I've been on the Pill, and a few naturally when I was a teen. A diagnosis of polycystic ovaries when I was 19, predating my liver disease/lupus diagnoses. IUD caused immense, months-long bleeding upon insertion.

She donned a blue plastic apron and signalled for me to hoist myself on to the bed. Two minutes later an ultrasound wand contraption was sailing its way up my vaginal canal. With her free hand, she was pointing to a black and white pixelated version of one of my ovaries on a nearby monitor.

"You see here," she circled what I could only describe as a mottled shadow on the screen. "You have lots of eggs. Plenty eggs. I count about 15 follicles there." I craned my neck at an unnatural angle from the bed, straining the tendons to see more shadows dancing around. I hummed in vague agreement but had absolutely no clue what I was even meant to be looking at. "Yes, you have a good egg count. An excellent egg count.[82]" I felt oddly proud of my ovaries. "You can redress now."

I shimmied back into my trousers and sat down by the desk again.

"With an egg count like this, you absolutely *would* be viable for freezing…" She clasped her hands together gently, leaning forward in her chair. "…if only you didn't have any of your other health problems."

I noticed for the first time that this doctor was likely only a few more years older than me. Her wedding ring sat quietly underneath a more ostentatious engagement diamond. I wondered if she had children.

She continued. "And we cannot neglect the fact that you do have multiple other very serious health conditions. You see, when we do a harvest for egg freezing, we will pump you full of hormones. Sometimes, and especially when women have as good an egg count as yourself, then what we might see happen, is something called *overstimulation*." She put the last word in finger parenthesis. I've learned that it's never normally positive news when a doctor brings out the finger parenthesis. "And this phenomenon can put a lot of pressure on your organs. And if your organs are already under a lot of pressure, or aren't functioning particularly well, this can sometimes be…" she glanced over quickly at the accompanying medical student in the room, "…fatal."

I puffed out my cheeks and raised my eyebrows. "Oh. Okay.

[82] This sounds almost Trump-ish in its exaggerated description – the best egg count the world has ever seen - but this was honestly what she described it as.

I see." My voice broke a tiny bit. *Don't cry. Be brave. It's fine.*

She looked at me pleadingly, as if willing me to not get too defeated. "It's not a *definite* 'no'."

"But it's a very risky '*yes*'. I understand."

*Well, duh, Kirsty. The sheer audacity of you to even think you might be considered viable for any of this normal woman stuff. Let's remind you once again of quite how ill you really are. You should be grateful for being alive, never mind thinking you might be able to go on to have a family.*

She cocked her head over to one side. "I'd like to raise it at our interdepartmental meeting. Get some other opinions first, before we can decide one way or another whether we would be happy to proceed with this."

It's funny how emotionless these it's-probably-going-to-be-bad-news-but-we-can't-completely-confirm-it-yet kind of appointments leave me. My strategy, I think, is to treat them like professional business meetings, wherein I go in with a poker face and leave remarkably serene. My emotions then catch up with my thoughts hours after exiting the appointment room, when I fall headfirst into an emotional breakdown.

It's not that I drive back home and then fall to my knees in floods of tears, banging on the walls like a wronged banshee, furious at the desperate unfairness of the world. I mean, I probably *could*, if I wanted to. But my emotional breakdowns are more a general overwhelming wave of morose blahness. They arrive with an invisible blow that knocks the wind out of my sails and reminds me, time and time again, that I'm not normal; I'm simply burning time before something else even more medically freaky happens.

Over the next few weeks, that turned into months, I pushed the fertility appointment to the back of my mind. I think I managed to do this because there was a tiny bit of hope that the fated interdepartmental meeting would miraculously decide that, actually, I might be able to have my eggs frozen. Additionally, around the same time, my oesophageal varices were getting progressively worse and needed more frequent banding. In short, I had bigger health fish to fry.

*Six months* later, in the gloominess of early January, I arrived home after a long day at work to find an NHS-branded letter on my doormat. The details of this two-page letter from the fertility clinic, addressed to my GP but cc'ing me in, declared that there was no safe way I could become pregnant in my current condition, using IVF or otherwise.

Eight paragraphs, typed ever-so-neatly in the NHS-issue font but without any attempt to reduce medical jargon or simplify terminology, explained at length all the ways in which my conditions were conspiring against me. Statistical probabilities were provided for various equally terrifying eventualities. Risks of egg harvesting were outlined, and mortality rates were quoted, culminating in the conclusion that pregnancy, either natural or via IVF, was not advised in my current state. Indeed, the faceless consortium confirmed, pregnancy would prove difficult even in a hypothetical post-transplant situation, as whilst some of the dangers regarding varices might not remain, I'd still be incredibly high risk with lupus and reliant on very heavy-duty immunosuppressant medication.

And then there was the final flourish: a throwaway sentence stating that, should I ever wish to be at a point where I would like to conceive, I would be best to get back in touch with the fertility team through my GP to discuss my options.

I re-read the letter to make sure I had understood correctly. It definitely sounded like I had no options remaining, really, unless I wanted spontaneous organ failure. I slid down onto the floor of my living room, back pressed tight against the radiator for warmth because my flat's central heating hadn't been on all day, and I cried. I cried for the version of me having to read that letter, alone. I cried for the little imaginary-cloud children who lived somewhere in my mind, and who suddenly evaporated back into the brain ether. I cried for my parents, to whom I couldn't provide a grandchild. I cried for any future partner I might have, and how they would need to also be aligned to not having children with me. And then, when I couldn't cry more because I felt stupid and my nose was fully blocked, I filed the letter into my arch binder of NHS letters.

Case closed. Whilst this was an abrupt end to my short-lived IVF 'journey', I believe it was the least painful way forwards in a losing game. That letter, callous as it seemed, was a definitive answer. I avoided the immense pain of miscarriages or invasive, drawn-out investigations. I saved myself the heartache, the physical scars and the financial strain of rounds and rounds of IVF which have such a devastating impact on many other ladies. Yes, I've felt the door of natural motherhood slam shut in my face without so much as a 'hello', but maybe that was the kindest way.

# ON BEING CHRONICALLY SCOTTISH

Mark Renton, protagonist of Irvine Welsh's *Trainspotting,* was not wrong when he declared it was "shite being Scottish". Existing in a land with minimal daylight during winter and apocalyptic cloud coverage during the months which the rest of the northern hemisphere refers to as 'summer', leads to not only sustained Vitamin D deficiency but a hardened psyche.

We Scots survive annual plagues of midges, being considered as outside of the British Isles for the purpose of furniture deliveries, and having only a handful of Waitrose branches in the entire country (yet, somehow, we survive). As such, we've learned to address life's challenges head on, with an optional six-foot claymore sword, tartan kilt and blue face paint.

I'm not *that* Scottish person who proudly swings a Saltire air freshener from the car mirror, or whose Spotify Wrapped is topped by *Auld Lang Syne.* Every cell of my soul cringes at the mere mention of *Outlander*, and my veins are not coursing with the neon nectar of Irn Bru. Despite my staunch anti-stereotype viewpoint, it's hard to deny that there are defining characteristics that bind Scots together.

Our resilience and bloody-mindedness, our historical ability to persevere through adversity, has passed down the generations. We did not let a lack of household electricity, running water and indoor toilets prevent us from inventing the pneumatic tyre and telephone. My ancestors would huddle together round fires drying herring in small smokehouses, or risk life and limb on the North Sea waves just to catch a living. Their robustness lives on not only in my sturdy cankles (jeans with anything slimmer than a bootcut are a no-no) but in my penchant for being fantastically stubborn.

As a people, Scots are renowned for their shrewdness, sarcasm, and self-depreciating humour, but it's (usually) offset by an enduring humility. Scots have a beleaguered but relentless appreciation for the small wins: an unsquashed Tunnocks teacake, or avoiding being swooped upon by teradactyl seagulls. It's this sense of Scottishness that, in a roundabout way, helps me cope.

Living with autoimmune disease is a bit like playing a relentless tennis match against an automatic ball thrower, where I spend most of my time batting away new problems, skidding across the court so as not to miss new symptoms, or contorting my backhand in order to keep everything ticking along safely. There are times when I reckon the volley is more or less under control, when I'm batting things away with relative ease. Other times, it feels like I've played the machine for six hours straight, only for it to be replaced by Andy Murray after a breakfast of Weetabix and two double espressos, with Federer chucking in some non-health related curveballs from the sidelines, too.

There's only so much a brain can deal with without melting. I often get to a stage where there are just so many things to worry about – and I still haven't quite learned the knack to not worry at all – that my mind simply cannot fit in any more anxiety. And that's the moment when, from the bottom of my brain, a Glaswegian (not sure why it's specifically Glaswegian, it's probably because mostly they're inherently funny and down-to-earth) voice pops up and says:

*"Aye, okay hen, it's a bit shite, but gonnae calm yoursel' down a bit?"*

The Scottishness in me saves myself from taking it all too seriously. More importantly, it prevents me from taking *myself* too seriously. After all, I hark from a country whose national income is sturdily supported by a three-humped dinosaur chilling in Loch Ness; our ability to take the piss is without limits.

Whilst it's tough being cheery, I find it's tougher to be miserable all the time. Despite our reputation for dourness, I think us Scots are, at heart, positive people. We like to see the good in others. Yes, we may moan like foghorns about how it's rained for 94 days straight in Glasgow, be a little rough round the edges, be averse to spending our hard-earned cash (trips to London become one long consecutive exclamation of '*How much*?!'), and not suffer fools gladly.

But much like our national flower[83], beneath the exterior of prickly thorns lies an innate…well, *beauty* probably isn't the right word, but certainly a *softness*. We have a unicorn as our national symbol. Years ago, we looked into the eyes of deepest, darkest winter, and said, feck this, let's have a big party every New Years' Eve followed by a swim the next day in the

---

[83] The thistle, just to avoid doubt.

freezing cold waters of the Firth of Forth, and call the whole spectacle 'Hogmanay'. Confronting general shittiness with a cheeriness is our national pastime.

We also have a deliciously dark sense of humour, which I use like a crutch. Sometimes things get so serious, so frightening, that the only way to cope without having a full-on meltdown is to make light of the whole situation and observe the absurdity of it all like the director of the Truman show. I have never quite got used to being a patient. To my mind, I'm just Kirsty, and the fact that all this is happening to me by some godforsaken unfortunate coincidence is a joke. A really shite joke, but a joke, nonetheless.

Above all, Scots are allergic to making a fuss. We casually discovered electricity, invented fridges, pedal bikes, kaleidoscopes, steam engines, colour photographs, caramel wafers and cloned the first sheep, but lo! If anyone was to point this out, we'd most likely pass it all off as no big deal. When someone tried to drive a jeep with propane gas into Glasgow airport, the retired Glaswegian fireman who calmly extinguished the resulting fire did so before going home for a shower, taking his wife out for dinner as planned, and neglecting to mention he averted a terrorist attack until she saw him on the television news. No drama.

My mother – for whom it must be emotionally wrenching to witness her child be ill, and for her to not be able to fix it – has never cried in front of me, never refused to listen to me moan, and is an incredibly steadfast presence waiting in the wings of each and every one of my medical dramas. She does so without complaining or making a song and dance about it.

My grandparents lost a baby girl when she was a few days old, but they never got compassionate leave from work, and 'counselling' may as well have been a foreign language in 1950s' rural Scotland. Instead, they never talked about her for over 50 years. Now, I'm not advocating this approach as anything near healthy, and I'm certainly not downplaying how much this must have affected my grandparents, but it just demonstrates that the family I've been brought up by are people who just…get on with it.

And it is precisely this sense of level-headedness that has been crucial to my ability to cope with what's been served up on my plate. Everyone has problems; it's all about how you choose to deal with them. To paraphrase Mark Renton: choose positivity. Choose taking the piss out of yourself a wee bit from time to time. Choose life.

# ON MENTAL HEALTH

It happens so easily, so insidiously, that I'm never quite prepared. Like an annoying mosquito, I bat away negative emotions into a nice wee 'think about this later' compartment of my psyche whenever the physical aspects of my condition take centre stage. *Poor mental health*, I tell myself, *won't kill me before a cirrhotic liver, aplastic anaemia, or kidney failure will.* During flares of my illness, I have limited energy, and this calls for a need to prioritise accordingly. I simply don't have the headspace to worry, or get angry, upset, or disappointed.

The biggest problem with this strategy, of course, is that the longer that 'think about this later' box is left with problematic emotions rotting inside, the more the leaching gases of unaddressed feelings expand, forcing the bolts on the box to buckle under the pressure. Then one day, when I'm totally unprepared, the box bursts open, unleashing its chaos in my relationships, my self-esteem, my work, and every other aspect of my life. And it usually takes a long time to clean it all back up again. Sometimes the stains never quite fade, and I always regret not tending to the emotional aspects earlier.

Mental health can often be overlooked when it comes to chronic illness. Society may well be awash with mental health lingo and social media channels rallying out the line that 'it's okay not to be okay', but what if you're never going to be 'okay' again? What happens when your body fundamentally changes the way it works?

In my experience, mental health is the elephant in the diagnosis room that is often ignored. The NHS is, I think, unequipped to automatically prescribe mental health support as a side serving to the main course of being told you have a lifelong health condition. Sure, it will happen for some patients, but certainly not all.

Learning to live with chronic issues is a mental burden. Chronically ill patients are not immune from divorce, bullying, redundancies, grief, or indeed any of life's shit sandwiches. Unfortunately, we have the additional crappy condiments of everything else I've explained in this book, all the while feeling unwell or in pain for a lot of the time *and* living in a world that is regrettably setup for able-bodied people.

This is the mental struggle that each one of us with chronic illness faces, to a greater or lesser extent, every day. The balance is incredibly fragile: even when things are going well, and your physical health is good, it only takes one bad 'life' blip for everything to easily fall apart again. Things always creep out of the woodwork. There came a point in my early 20s where it dawned on me that I was never again going to be able to *not* worry to some extent about my health.

There will always remain a low-level anxiety in the background, and the list of 'things I've worried about that have never actually materialised' could be a book franchise all on its own. But how best to manage it all without needing to grab the nearest paper bag and start controlled breathing exercises to stave off panic?

I'm not very good at proactively looking after my mental health. I think I get away with it because, generally speaking, I'm genetically prone to being positive and upbeat, and don't get 'down' too easily. Nonetheless, I always forget to make notes in preparation for the nerve-racking times when my liver function tests go awry. What's more, as demonstrated by my November 2002 production of 'Alfie's Adventures in Ancient Egypt' (an I.P.-infringing am-dram interpretation of a Tesco kids' book that I produced, directed, recorded, costume-designed, sound-checked and co-starred in with my sister), I'm gifted at putting on a good show.

I compartmentalise my personality like a boss. Thing is, I'm not sure who I do this for: other people, or myself. Sometimes I'm not even sure which version of me is the real Slim Shady. I am one person (serious, stoic and rational) to my doctors, and another (emotional, garrulous and vulnerable) to my family and friends. But being able to switch between these versions of me is, I think, part of my coping strategy; I need a balance of the two in order to keep it all together.

I can paint on a MAC Ruby Woo smile and pretend everything is fine. It's not just me who's guilty of doing this; the world runs on the ability of a subset of the population to put on a brave face whilst silently crying into the abyss of their soul. Sometimes, it's good to keep calm and carry on. But other times, it winds up being more toxic than a nuclear waste leak.

There have been two periods in my life when I've

recognised that I'm feeling so unconnected to myself that I've asked for help from a clinical psychologist. The first time was four months after being diagnosed with liver disease, and the second was in the weeks after I received the letter from the fertility clinic ruling out biological motherhood in my current circumstances.

It's interesting to note that the times when I've sought professional help both relate to grieving a version of my life that I won't lead: firstly, the life without a liver disease and, more recently, the life where I could have had biological children. Whilst I'm used to illness involving lots of micro-grieving – missed holidays due to illness, missed weddings because of gastritis, missed moments of youthful recklessness – these losses are ultimately surmountable. They come, they're felt, and they fade with the passing of time. But this grief felt more seismic.

On reflection, this pain, the grief, is the price paid for being human, for being alive and for having feelings. I'd be more concerned if I managed to turbo-charge through such big shifts *without* being emotionally ransacked. During these times, I've not been 'sad', or 'down'. I've been mentally *numb*. Numb, as though the chemicals that would normally work to give me emotions have decided to go full-on French and strike, leaving a flaming Fiat 500 carcass in their wake. Numb, as though I'm in self-protection mode because the battery in my soul short-circuited.

Everyday life became overcast with a wash of greyscale. There were moments – zoning out at work meetings, or whilst queueing at the self-scanners in Sainsbury's – when I had an overriding, out-of-nowhere, need to cry. But along with these urges to break into tears, I simultaneously felt an overpowering urge *not to*, because if I did, I was afraid that I might not be able to stop. Sometimes I felt frozen. Other times I felt like everything was so out of control and unmanageable and overwhelming, and my chest ached as though it physically needed to cave in.

"It's like, I'll be walking down the street on my way to meet a friend, or go to a lecture, and I'll just want to cry," I explained, post cirrhosis-diagnosis, how I felt to a sympathetic GP at the university health centre. "And I don't think it's normal to cry for an hour on the phone to your mum every single night, either."

"Oh, Kirsty," she grimaced. "I'm so sorry. But I don't think you're clinically depressed. I think, instead, what you're going through is a completely normal reaction to being diagnosed with a serious health condition." I nodded, understanding that my feelings were a response to my situation, but not really wanting her to confirm that there was no easy escape other than to just work through this feeling. She continued. "And I don't want to prescribe antidepressants. Not only would they be quite bad for your liver, but also because I don't actually think that would help you feel any better."

The most painful part, the part that no medicine and no amount of talking therapy could help with, was that I felt so incredibly helpless. Until that point, I had never really encountered any big life challenge. I'd never needed to deploy the heavy-duty machines stocked up in my emotional toolkit. Suddenly, I was finding that my inability to move forward was both a novel experience and a terrifying prospect.

"Everything seems so *pointless*," I recall telling my liver doctor, a few weeks after that GP appointment. We were in the same room where he told me I had cirrhosis just six months prior. "Like, what's the point in even trying to do well, trying to complete my degree to get a good job, when I feel I've already tripped over at the very first hurdle in life?"

He took his glasses off and pinched the bridge of his nose. "I must admit, I didn't realise you were struggling. You appeared to me to be coping with it all very well. But then again, I suppose I only see one side of things."

"Yeah. Well, I'm not really managing very well." I pulled my mouth to one side in a grimace, biting the inside of my mouth as a comfort mechanism. I doubted he was the only one I'd fooled. If you had taken a survey of the people with whom I interacted over these periods, I'd bet they would all say I seemed absolutely normal. Happy, even. "I think I might just give it all up."

He looked at me.

"Uni, I mean. Give up uni," I clarified.

"I don't think it's a good idea to give up your studies, Kirsty." His gentle chastisement stung a little. I knew he was right, but I wanted just a moment to push back against all that was happening. To threaten to be a rebel, without actually going through with it.

"But does it ever get any better? Will this ever get easier to deal with?" I don't know what I was expecting him to say. Maybe I wanted him to morph into Mystic Meg.

"The only thing I can recommend, from other patients' experiences, is to give it time. You are still very early on in your diagnosis. You might feel differently in the future."

Again, he was right. I believe, clichéd as it is, that time is one of the best healers. The distance from painful events, the benefit of hindsight, the experience of living with a condition and understanding the reality of its ups and downs, the learnings and the wisdom and the self-confidence gained from each rollercoaster dip, is a form of therapy in itself. Maybe it was more a lack of general life experience that made it particularly difficult to process this first bout of depression when I was first diagnosed.

But time can't be the only therapy. For me, cognitive behavioural therapy with a psychologist has helped the processing of my feelings, particularly during more difficult periods. Being able to articulate my thoughts to a neutral party forces a deeper, more valuable level of self-reflection. Problems that I ruminate over in my head often don't seem so terrifying when I explain them aloud.

I've been guilty of walking into an appointment assuming that the psychiatrist is going to solve everything like a paracetamol fixing a headache. Imagine my disappointment, then, when I've left therapy sessions feeling *worse* than I did going in. It's not a golden bullet, but it does help to ground me in those moments where things all get a bit too much.

But even when things are relatively stable from a health perspective, and I'm not feeling disconnected from myself, there is low-level anxiety that exists along with my conditions. It winds up being something of a continuous game of moving the goal posts. Just when one aspect of my health seems manageable or stable, it always feels like something else in my life will go berserk. It's a never-ending battle, and one which I have limited control over.

I am pretty open about my health issues. Indeed, I probably overshare; the line between what is and is not socially acceptable becomes blurred after you've had to describe your rectal bleeding to the GP. Being open helps me to talk about my feelings more easily. And I talk *a lot.* With my parents. With my sister. With my friends and my workmates and with people in online support groups. With Poppy, my parents' labrador, who always thinks I'm right.

I'll ask for advice from these same groups, but nobody (not even me) can fully understand all the intricacies of my health conditions. Whilst talking about physical and mental health is far more commonplace than ever before, there are still some details of my medical problems – persistent warts, mouth ulcers, or colitis, for example – which I just wouldn't broach on a coffee date with my pals.

So whilst having a support network is essential, it sometimes isn't enough. To lessen my health anxiety, I try to learn the science behind my conditions. A bit of knowledge (but not *too* much) is power. I find it also helps me to ask pertinent questions and feel empowered in making informed decisions about my health. I read medical journals, and blogs, and BMJ press releases, and Liver Anatomy books. I read about other liver diseases and research the latest news about medicines for autoimmune conditions.

Every so often I'll read something that I find enlightening. In my mid-20s, I finally came across Viktor Frankl's 'Man's Search for Meaning'. Frankl who was a prisoner in a concentration camp during the Holocaust, who survived and went on to become a leading psychologist who developed the concept of 'logotherapy'. This form of psychotherapy is underpinned by the notion that, as humans, we are driven to search for purpose in life, and finding this meaning is essential for wellbeing (even in adverse circumstances).[lxxiv] Frankl emphasised that individuals are never entirely without freedom of choice over their attitudes:

*"Everything can be taken from a man but one thing: the last of the human freedoms—to choose one's attitude in any given set of circumstances, to choose one's own way."*[lxxv]

At the risk of sounding like a pretentious twit (and who are we kidding, it's probably clear by now that I am one of the most pretentious but well-meaning twits), I'm also a big fan of reading up on Stoic philosophy. Stoicism encourages living life in accordance with various virtues (namely wisdom, justice, courage and moderation). One of its core concepts is that much of what happens in life is external to the remit of our personal control and should be accepted as such. According to Epictetus, one of the most famous Stoics:

*"We cannot choose our circumstances, but we can always choose how to interpret these situations and how to react to them."*

It takes a lot of effort, but I try to scrutinise my perspective on circumstances in life and remain laser-focussed on keeping a positive spin on them. I try to release negative thoughts into the ether. Essentially, I pour my energy into the parts of life over which I have control.

For example, it took me a long time to realise that I can't control the results of my blood tests. I can't control when my liver will start failing. I can't control how long I might wait for a liver transplant. Of course, it *is* within my control to live as healthily as possible in the meantime (by eating well, getting enough sleep, keep taking my drugs, and so on), but beyond that, it's out of my hands. Therefore, according to Stoicism, there's no point stressing about these things. I focus on making the most of the day ahead and trust that, if and when my liver does start failing, I will have the strength and courage to deal with that situation at that time.

Over the years, I've learned to create a (fairly massive) space for my health-related anxieties in the car park of my mind. I'm no Seneca[84], but I now approach problems with an ability to pretty quickly determine which elements are outside my sphere of control. After I've subjected a situation to the "is-this-in-my-circle-of-influence" litmus test, I'll park any concerns whilst resuming my daily life.

It's not a case of digging my head in the sand, or being in denial of my reality, but rather knowing how to apportion the right amount of time and emotion to the worry. Life is too short to let my illness – and thoughts about my illness – consume my psyche.

It's far easier said than done, of course, when chronic illness casts its shadow in almost every aspect of life. I still tend to overthink things with my rampant imagination. It is very easy to get caught up in a tornado of 'what if' thought experiments, and it takes significant effort to stop negative cycles and refocus, time and time again, on the aspects I can control.

Interestingly, however, I find that if I am consumed by negative thoughts, then it is generally an indication that my physical health is in good shape. For when I'm seriously ill, all my energy is funnelled into getting physically better. When my reserves are solely dedicated to staying alive, it's a bit easier to deal with, because the 'noise' of everyday life problems is filtered out.

Another key factor in improving my moods has been movement. Obviously, this is super difficult if you're in a lot

[84] One of the original Stoic philosophers.

of pain or shitting the equivalent of three meals out your backside for days on end, but I find even a little bit of gentle exercise is great for both my physical and mental health. I'm by no means pumping iron until the cows come home, but even getting out for a short walk leaves me in a much better mood.

Thing is, even if I didn't have a liver condition, I'm pretty sure there would be something else that I would fixate on as the 'problem' in my life. The key, I think, lies in learning to live with the uncertainty and the imperfection. To understand that there will probably be times in the future when I will feel numb again, but also times when I'll be happy. And I want to embrace it all, because I think that is what it means to fully live my life.

# ON OUR NHS

There are three steadfast pillars underpinning British society which are immune to all criticism:

1. David Attenborough documentaries

2. Cups of tea

3. The National Health Service.

The first two need no explanation – and if anyone disagrees, I'm sorry, but we can't be friends – so let us concentrate instead on the third. I'll begin with a positive attitude because the NHS, God love it, is the reason I'm alive. Indeed, it's the reason most of us Brits are here, unless you were posh enough to be privately pushed out at the Lindo Wing. It never fails to blow my mind that, before the NHS was established, people had to pay to see doctors and that childbirth would be more of a cross-your-fingers-and-pray-for-your-cervix situation.

The NHS has defended me from: measles, mumps, rubella,

polio, HPV, TB, flu, pneumonia, meningitis, hepatitis A and B, and Covid. It has provided resources to: correct my astigmatism aged five, avoid pregnancy, diagnose my faulty immune system, check my liver for cancer tumours twice a year, stop internal bleeding, check that I don't have varices that will bleed in the same way again, and help me face the world with three plastic wigs every year.

The best bit of all? This has been free for me at the point of use. The NHS is *the* reason I can enjoy the lifestyle I have today. If I lived in, say, America, I'd likely be bankrupt, uninsurable, or dead – perhaps all three. Which is all to say that I'm the NHS's number one fan. I really love it. I would nominate each person working for the NHS for an MBE sooner than you can say *celebrity personalities who don't deserve recognition.*

It pains me, then, to admit that the NHS is not the poster boy for healthcare. I'm no expert in the management of the service, and I don't know the details of the financials nor understand the extent of red tape that strangles the bureaucratic behemoth it has become. But I have experience of being the end customer, and I'm here to say that the service provided by the NHS is sometimes sub-standard.

Firstly, there's the technology. The staff use IT systems dating from when Bill Gates was still running Silicon Valley. I've spent precious minutes sitting in silence next to a GP whilst we both wait for a page of NICE guidance to crank up on the screen, pixel by pixel. Appointment times are routinely sent out by letter. More or less everything is conducted via phone calls, and with this comes a Magna Carta of confidentiality rules that often get in the way of efficient communication.

Talking of communication: it very often seems to be non-existent between different health boards, between GPs and consultants, between different consultants, and between the NHS and the patient. Patients with complex conditions needing help across several departments soon learn that there is a need to be able to join dots between admin teams in order to keep momentum. The NHS is like a huge cruise ship that moves nowhere fast, and its inner workings are labyrinthine in nature. Trying to push things through the right channels is a challenge.[85] Some trusts have apps, but there's no consistency between health boards. The NHS is, at the end of the day, like every other workplace. There is inefficiency, there is incompetence, and there is whopping mismanagement.

Yet when it works, the NHS is an incredible service comprising some amazing people who genuinely care and want to do the best for patients. People like the porter who gave me six additional sachets of contraband ketchup to have with my chips, or the endoscopist whose gently reassuring stroke of my hand after injecting propofol into its cannula gave me comfort whilst I counted down the 20 seconds for the sedative to take effect.

But all this runs on a hell of a lot of goodwill, and over the years I sense that this goodwill is fast on the burnout. The goodwill shouldn't involve nurses having to take blood pressure in freezing rooms with half-broken windowpanes, or consultants having to deliver life-changing news to patients whilst sat in airless and windowless side-rooms.

How to fix it? I'm not in any kind of position to advise, only to comment from the sidelines that I've been on the receiving

---

85 Which, of course, raises the question about how well patients who cannot advocate for themselves are served by the NHS.

end of a lot of inefficiency and poor communication. From my limited experience of 'improvement initiatives' in my own workplaces, I would cast a massive side-eye on paying astronomical sums of money to 'consultants' from 'management consultancies'. I've seen far too many of these cowboys spit out ineffectual nonsense before riding off into the sunset, never have to face the carnage they leave behind.

Is it possible to strive for better ways of working within such a complex organisation? I'm a realistic optimist, so I'd like to think that, yes, we can. *How* we do this, I'm not sure, but we must strive to maintain a health service we can be proud of for generations to come.

# ON GLOBAL PANDEMICS

One Friday night in January 2020, nestled in the nook of my parents' settee and watching the 10 o'clock news bulletin (wild, I know), my ears pricked up at the leading story. A new virus was sweeping its way across mainland China. There had been multiple deaths. All markets in a city called Wuhan had been shut down. China was entering a draconian-sounding lockdown. *Classic China*, I thought. *Totalitarianism 101*. It was probably for the best, given the size of their population. Still, it all seemed a bit heavy-handed.

This wasn't the first contagion outbreak since I officially joined the ranks of the immunocompromised. The avian flu in 2015 withered away into retirement after providing a fortnight of headline fodder. But this new coronavirus sounded like it had the potential to get quite bad. I pulled a face at my then-74-year-old father on the opposite sofa.

"What if *that*," I nodded to the VT of a biohazard-suited doctor half-jogging down an overcrowded hospital ward in Wuhan, "makes its way over *here*?"

Dad swirled the dregs of his wine and adjusted the seal-fresh clip on his bag of crisps. "All this will blow over. Mark. My. Words. I've seen this type of thing many times before. Don't worry about it."

"I think this one is different, though, Dad. They're locking down entire cities in China. Like, *millions* of people." I pointed at the pie charts on screen which a graphics team had clearly spent much time labouring over.

"Yes, but..." he sighed, reaching for the remote. "They're never going to ask *us* to stay inside. They can't. We can't stop the world for a virus. Come on. Let's watch something else."

Before long, the news reports escalated incrementally in their seriousness. Leaked medical stories of Wuhan emergency rooms were surfacing on Twitter. Antibacterial hand gel sold out in all branches of Boots, forcing people to Google how to concoct an alcohol-based alternative. Despite trying to maintain a façade of normality at work, with us all logging in to our emails and going through the motions, it was becoming undeniable that something was very amiss. There was a nervous energy about the office. Jokes-that-weren't-really-jokes were doing the rounds, talking about working from home for a month or, at a push, two.

Nobody was really paying attention in meetings, preferring instead to refresh BBC News every five minutes for some kind of formal direction from Government. International audits were postponed indefinitely, and I was second-guessing every sneeze within a two-metre radius of my desk. A colleague had recently returned from Dubai and said that the airports weren't taking any real measures to prevent infection on the planes. I moved my seat away from him when he started sniffling.

My boss pulled me aside one day and gave me permission to log in from home if it made me feel more comfortable. Friday the 13th of March 2020 was the last day I worked in an office for the next three years.

Exactly one week later, I switched on my telly to watch Boris Johnson issue a dystopian state address. Government (the people who we elect to create the rules of society) were asking us to stay inside to prevent the spread of Covid-19. Not so much a polite request, but a formal, legally binding order.

Everywhere was closing doors. Not just the fun places like cinemas and theatres, but schools, opticians, dentists, and care homes. Hospital appointments were cancelled unless critical. We sleepwalked into a real-life episode of Black Mirror. Even better, due to my winning combination of i) prolonged steroid use, ii) multiple immunosuppressive therapies and iii) severe liver disease, I fell into the bucket of being *extremely clinically vulnerable.*[86] Ding-ding-ding!

Like millions of others throughout the country, a letter from Downing Street dropped through my door a few days later. Unlike millions of others, though, I also went on to receive no fewer than *six* letters from a combination of the Scottish Chief Medical Officer, Scottish Deputy First Minister, Scottish First Minister, and Scottish Health Secretary. All the letters informed me in various terms that, because I was at most risk of getting seriously ill from this virus, I needed to STAY. THE. FUCK. INSIDE. (And then, in smaller print: for-at-least-12-weeks-but-maybe-longer-depending-on-reassessment.) It was a potent reminder of just how ill I really am. How precarious my health really is. You think you're normal, Kirsty? Ha! Think

---

[86] The tagline nobody will ever use on a Tinder profile.

again. We're going to keep you inside so you can have plenty of time, in isolation, to mull over just how seriously, freakishly *ab*normal you actually are.

12 weeks sounded just a little *too* convenient. It felt as though someone at the Health Committee meeting had initially suggested three (a pleasing aesthetic, but realistically too short a timeframe) or perhaps the lucky seven (best avoid anything Chinese-related), before an Oxbridge-educated ministerial busybody had a brainwave, remembering the disciples at the Last Supper before gingerly raising a hand and proffering a "12? Shall we go with 12? Worked for Jesus, didn't it?"

Besides, it didn't take a degree in immunology to work out that viruses wouldn't be contained in 12 paltry weeks. I pored over countless articles about how the only escape out of the lockdowns would be through modern medical interventions and vaccines. Not herd immunity, not start-stop lockdowns, but pure, cold science. Having dabbled in pharmaceuticals, I knew that vaccines were subject to the tightest of all regulatory requirements; there were so many hoops to jump through, so many trials to conduct. I knew that it would normally take years of work to demonstrate safety and efficacy, and so I was mentally gearing myself up to bid adieu to my youth and welcome in a years-long hiatus of my life.

It sounds bleak, and it was, to an extent. Until that point, I lived my life as fully as possible, keeping busy and enjoying every moment, knowing that my health was never guaranteed. I became frustrated that despite feeling well, I was looking at a future of being forced to waste precious time being inside and alone. There were moments where it dawned on me that other, 'healthy' people my age would most likely be able to rejoin 'normal' life faster than me.

Not leaving my flat seemed excessive given that a grand total of four people would pass my window every day, but I am nothing if not a true conformist. I vowed to the assorted health secretaries that my foot would not pass the threshold of my flat…which was all fine and dandy until my bins needed to be taken out. And then I figured that if I had taken the mortal risk to put bin bags out, I might as well go for a bit of a walk down the street. The 12 weeks of hardcore Castaway-existence turned into seven days of not leaving my flat at all, followed by months of solo walks at lunch and in the evenings.

Bizarrely, I look back on summer 2020 somewhat fondly. There were many people for whom the lockdowns were extremely debilitating, but I was fortunate to have been in a comfortable flat, with job security, an ability to work remotely and, most importantly, family who lived locally. Friends would show their support through quiet acts of love like flatpack bouquets and DIY clay rainbow kits that would drop through my letterbox.

Naturally, there were moments of catastrophising worst-case scenarios: what if I needed a transplant during this time (all non-emergency transplants were cancelled), or what if my medicines stopped manufacturing, or what if the hospitals went into meltdown and we became an apocalyptic state? What if there was rioting in the streets and people started looting and there was a global food shortage? What if we never found a treatment or vaccine?

But equally, there was a simplicity to my lockdown era. I wasn't progressing in life, but it felt like nobody else was, either. There was no competition to be hitting life's milestones. We were all facing a new, unknown future where those old milestones might never again apply.

In some ways, I felt that the pandemic highlighted the diversity of the clinically vulnerable group, as if to say: *the vulnerable walk amongst us! They're not just in care homes or stuck in high dependency units!* Some people started to better understand what normal life was like for immunocompromised people, too. *See*, I thought, watching people load up on antibacterial hand gel and cough into the crooks of their arms, *this is a glimpse into the anxiety levels with which I've lived for years: a constant, rumbling fear when someone sneezes or coughs or smears their germs across a door handle which you're about to touch*. The quirks which had become my everyday practice – jerking a jacket arm over my hand before touching lift buttons or avoiding the air stream of someone who's just sneezed – suddenly wound up in the everyday repertoire of Joe Public.

Mundane things that I took for granted before Covid re-established a new value. Venturing outside my hometown seemed like an exotic treat; I recall going to hospital for an IUD removal, having not had a face-to-face appointment for months, and feeling like I was going abroad. My routine – of getting up, doing Joe Wicks' online exercise videos, having breakfast, and then going to work online, before trying to maximise time in the evenings by practicing guitar or reading a book – felt monastic but also mildly romantic. Yet whilst I carved out this new normality, there were still moments where I wondered what lay ahead.

How long would I be kept inside, unable to join group events? Indeed, would it ever again be safe for me to do so? Moreover, how did I ever feel safe being in groups of big people before? It was suddenly unbelievable that there hadn't been more outbreaks of epidemics like Covid previously, given the scale of globalisation. Would I ever be able to meet anyone again without a PCR test beforehand? Surely, they couldn't leave the severely immunocompromised to stay in and avoid people forever, right? *Right?*

Nothing felt secure anymore, but then I realised nothing was ever secure before, either. It was such a big worry and one that had no forthcoming answers or elements within my control, that I soon decided to stop giving it too much thought in order to avoid exploding with anxiety. The only option, I felt, was to just get on with it.

Living alone meant I easily avoided human contact, the only exception being when I had to get bloods taken. A nurse, fully decked out in full-blown PPE, visited my house as it was deemed too risky for me to visit a health centre. I didn't actually sit with another non-PPE-ed human (my Mum) in the same room for a few months after lockdown started.

All things concerned, my Covid position could have been a lot worse, but a lot of people seemed to think that it must have been awful being alone for that length of time. Perhaps it's a reflection of my introversion that I didn't mind that it was just me, myself, and I. It felt safer. I was in control. I even viewed the solitude as a challenge to make the most of; being unable to travel, I decided that each weekend would consist of virtual visits to different cities. One weekend, for example, the theme was Paris, so I donned a Breton top, baked baguettes, and had croissants for breakfast whilst doing a virtual tour of the Musee D'Orsay. (I know, I'm a geek.)

Yet Covid is the gift that keeps giving, and its side-effects have seeped surreptitiously like a poison ivy over the nation's bones. There is, understandably, a fatigued weariness in the medical profession. In a system which operates largely owing to the goodwill of medical staff from the lowest to the top ranks, it sometimes feels like the tap is running dry. There is only so much that humans can deal with, and I feel the NHS system is buckling under the immense strain it's borne for too many years.

And the effects ripple outside of medical spheres, too. What was initially an equaliser – we were all forced into a new reality where our ability to continue life as before lockdown was substantially disrupted – soon turned into a force for heightened inequality. Covid has ripped apart our social fibres and repatched them in a mismatched pattern. The rich got richer, the poor got poorer.

Whilst people like me, already facing challenging health conditions, stayed indoors and were prepared to put a pause on their life for as long as it took, our Cabinet felt it was fitting to throw champagne-fuelled garden parties. Some people argue that this whole debacle was blown out of proportion, that it was only a few drinks, that our Prime Minister and his cabal deserved to have time to relax. My response to those people is that Boris Johnson wouldn't know personal sacrifice if it came and hit him in the face.

There was absolutely nothing 'equal' in our collective experience of the pandemic, and I feel it has only served to accelerate the rate of divergence between our society's 'haves' and 'have-nots'. Some people – the ones, you'll recall, who we elected to make the rules – thought, and undoubtedly continue to think, that those very same rules don't apply to them.

To properly address the lasting effects, whatever they may be, perhaps we first need to acknowledge the sacrifice that most of the population made for our country. Each generation relinquished aspects of their life to protect the greater society. Most of us played by the rules; we didn't visit dying relatives, we gave birth alone on distanced labour wards, with midwives behind PPE screens. We watched, through low-pixel cameras with microphones unprotected from blasts of Arctic winds, friends getting married in gardens. We dialled into Teams calls from cluttered bedrooms. We used our allocated exercise hour to walk to Tesco, only to realise we forgot a mask, returning the next day to march down aisles anticlockwise and in single file. We stayed in mould-ridden flats with three children under the age of eight who were left to learn how to write from two hours' worth of lessons on iPads.

*That's* sacrifice. And how do we mark it collectively? We don't. It feels like the whole era has been swept under the sleaze-stained carpet of Westminster. An act of remembrance might serve to re-emphasise some of the collective lessons learned from the pandemic. It might serve as a testament to the importance of public health, or how it was science that saved the day when it came to Covid. After all, it was test tubes, not tinfoil hats, that allowed us to return to something vaguely reminiscent of normal life.

Even now, half a decade after the start of the pandemic, there remain many clinically vulnerable people who feel too anxious to go to crowded places or use public transport in fear of catching Covid. Others won't venture out without a mask, and even when they do, will be ridiculed for doing so. I think it boils down to a personal evaluation of risk. I have had Covid three times now and haven't suffered too badly as a result, so would therefore risk re-catching the virus (even with the potential for added complications due to long Covid) rather than risk losing years of my life hiding inside.

But of course, the risk balance is always liable to change, and what is acceptable to one person might not be the same evaluation as another.

We never know what other people are going through, but we can be sure that the impacts of Covid didn't end at the lifting of the lockdown. I am very fearful that the way we navigated the Covid pandemic will have a negative impact on the way we navigate future pandemics, and what that will mean for the clinically vulnerable. The invisible scars of the pandemic remain, more deeply on some than on others, and it is so important that they are not forgotten.

# ONWARDS

*"Hope for the best, prepare for the worst"*

*Neville Chamberlain*

"And finally, have you ever been notified of being at risk of Mad Cow Disease by the Scottish Government?" The nurse asked as he shook a delightfully emo fringe off his eyes. He held a pen above the one final checkbox on the questionnaire affixed to his clipboard. "It's just, we have to ask all patients before they get endoscopies. It's actually not unheard-of round this area."

I hesitated in my response, trying to work out if I was playing to a receptive crowd. Did Oban Hospital staff have a sense of humour? Judging by the 1970s-style patterns on the curtains, they certainly had a sense of humour when it came to interior design. "Not to my knowledge. But I guess that's up for debate."

I laughed (ha! As if, by joking, I could convince myself that

I was looking forward to being wheeled through for yet another endoscopy), he laughed (ha-ha! As if nobody had ever made that awful joke before), and Mum laughed (ha-ha-ha! As if it wasn't gut-wrenching to say goodbye to your daughter and have to pray that, when you pick her up again in an hour, none of the advertised risks of the procedure have actually happened).

Then he slid a cannula into the back of my hand (the crooks of both elbows, where the needle would otherwise go, were a sorry spectrum of purple and green bruises from previous blood draws) and walked me through to the endoscopy 'suite' for what would end up being my fourth round of banding within nine months. This was possibly the most I had ever needed in that timeframe. Therein lies the rub: despite me doing everything I possibly can to keep healthy, I'm merely delaying the inevitable. My liver will ultimately wind up failing.

I've been able to somewhat adapt my life around that expectation, but over the years, I feel like I'm in a weird purgatory. I'm *too well* to require a transplant assessment, but I'm still suffering from some of the (potentially lethal) symptoms of advanced liver disease. The risks of transplant surgery currently outweigh the risks of *not* transplanting, but that balance may switch fairly rapidly at any point in my future.

More recently, I have been encountering more and more signs that my liver is unhappily grumbling away under the surface, like an organ version of the super caldera at Yellowstone National Park. Sometimes it's innocuous symptoms such as more spider veins on my face and hands, or I'll spy little trails of platelet bruises on my arms with no apparent cause, or have nosebleeds during the night which wake me up just in time to run to the bathroom to plug the stream with tissue.

Then there are the more concerning symptoms: waking up some mornings to swollen veins bulging around my belly button. Night sweats. Having the slightest tinge of yellow skin when I wake up from a nap, or ultrasound scans showing more and more pockets of fluid chilling out in my abdomen. The immunosuppressive effect pokes its head into the party from time to time, too – an ever-lovely reminder that it's always going to be lurking in the shadows.

There are the outbreaks of shingles or random rashes on my back, warts that wouldn't look out of place on the *Creature from the Black Lagoon*, fortnightly bouts of diarrhoea or random, debilitating stomach cramps. The steroids give way to spontaneous episodes of thrush and UTIs, or elevated levels of EBV and CMV[87] viral loads, or bloodshot eyes and styes, cracked skin and weakened bones.

These are all drip-drip reminders that my body is keeping many plates spinning internally but is liable to spontaneous failure. Sometimes I imagine myself to be in a slow-motion car crash where the freeze frames are shifting one to the next, but more quickly with each passing year. I just don't know when the crunch point is going to be, or how much suffering I'll have to endure in the meantime.

Even post-crunch point, if I'm lucky enough to have a liver transplant[88], it's not all rainbows and sunshine. My immune system is liable to start attacking *that* liver, too, causing AIH in the new organ. If everything goes to plan (and it often doesn't),

---

[87] Epstein-Barr virus (EBV) and Cytomegalovirus (CMV) are two viral infections that are relatively common and treatable in healthy people, but potentially dangerous to the immunosuppressed. EBV can cause glandular fever.

[88] Contrary to popular belief, livers fit for transplant are not easy to come by, and the waiting list is very long.

liver transplantation is a heavy-duty operation – both physiologically and emotionally – with months-long recovery and lifelong implications. Overarching all this, my lupus will remain. Transplant or not, there's no golden bullet cure to any of this. And *that's* scary.

One suffocatingly warm May afternoon, straight after my traumatising final Honours exam, I ventured out with pals to the Student Union to celebrate the anticlimactic end of our university careers. We discussed our post-graduation plans. My friends chatted excitedly about what their summers held in store: an internship at a publishing house in London, backpacking round Europe, jetting off to Australia, a graduate job at an accountancy firm.

"It's so exciting, isn't it? The not knowing what's going to happen next. Like, your life could quite possibly take on any direction from here on in. Endless opportunities ahead," one of the girls mused as she reached across the table to dip a curly fry into our little pot of ketchup.

I half-heartedly hummed in agreement whilst trying hard to avoid having a full-on anxiety breakdown at the table. First and foremost, I had successfully convinced myself in the two hours since we poured out of the exam hall that I had bombed the organic chemistry paper (because *of course* that carbon couldn't have formed a six-way pi bond in question 8). But moreover, the concept of not knowing what I was doing next, not having even a whiff of a pencilled-in plan, for the very first time in my life was genuinely terrifying.

Whilst it felt like everyone else at least had freedom with which to *explore* their options, I wasn't sure how much longer I'd have a functioning liver. At the stage in life when I should arguably have felt like the whole world was for the taking, when the opportunities I'd worked for began to materialise, it had never felt more closed off.

And whilst I look back now and think, *gah, I shouldn't have worried so much*, hindsight is a wonderful thing. I don't ever regret being more cautious, or taking the safer options, because I think it's helped me to escape a lot of the worst liver disease symptoms for as long as I have. Whilst I've converted, to some extent, that fear of the unknown into motivation to do things whilst I'm able, there is an omniscient sense of creeping mortality at the back of my mind. There is no inbuilt countdown timer for when my liver might fail, or my drugs might stop working, or when my next flare might be, and that means I can't plan. Being comfortable in that uncomfortableness, as a control freak, is very difficult and probably not something I'll ever fully accept.

Birthdays, parties, weekend plans – things that other people normally look forward to – come loaded with a degree of stress. Holidays, too, are often more stress than they're worth. How would I cope with being dramatically ill abroad, having to explain my medical history through Google translate? What if I get queried at security with my stash of prednisone, and forget to take a prescription slip to prove that I'm not, in fact, Pablo Escobar? I'm usually able to override these thoughts by telling myself the risk is worth the life experience; it's better to just take life as it comes and try to enjoy the experiences as they happen.

What is my greatest fear of all? I don't think it's a fear of death, *per se*. No, my fear is wrapped up in knowing that my health is going to have to get worse before it can get better. When my liver does give up the gun, it might be a slow decline, having the things I enjoy about my life right now be stripped away, one by one, over years, waiting for a liver to be available to transplant…or it might be a rapid descent, suffering some of the most gnarly complications of advanced liver disease. I'm not sure which version would be worse.

As mentioned in a previous chapter, worsening liver disease can sometimes cause a condition called hepatic encephalopathy. A quick reminder: this is when the toxins in your blood aren't cleared properly by your liver and instead make their way into your brain, causing undesirable (albeit usually temporary, if treated quickly) character changes and brain damage. The prospect of this one condition, above all the others[89], is what freaks me out the most. I pride myself on being cheery; I love my wee internal narrative that witters on, and my ability to think rationally and crack jokes. And this is why I am shit-scared about changes to my personality from some of these rare, but not unimaginable, complications.

There are enormous challenges in my road ahead. Being assessed for transplantation would unlock new levels of anxiety ranging from the not knowing whether a match would be found in sufficient time, to the crushing guilt involved with the implicit understanding that, essentially, someone will have to die in order for me to live. A transplant will only ever be a treatment that allows me to live longer. It is not a cure.

Yet as much as I might think that acting out the worst-case prognosis scenarios in my imagination will help prepare me for all conceivable eventualities, it doesn't. In my experience, the things I've been most affected by, that have substantially changed the course of my life, are the things I never even considered in my triple-locked backup plans.

---

[89] And let's be clear: there are probably lots of complications I am blissfully unaware of, too.

Sure, I could hole myself up in a Wifi-less bothy somewhere north of Ullapool, refusing all social contact and shaking a translucent fist at the rain-filled sky. I could spend my days cursing the cruel hand dealt to me in life's game of cards and bemoaning all the things that I can't do (or that are endlessly more difficult to do) because of my chronic illnesses. But such an attitude serves nobody any good in the longer term. A life of spite and negativity is not one that I choose to lead; I owe it to myself to *try* to be happy.

Every single person on this planet faces some level of difficult situations. Even Taylor Swift, whilst winning in the wealth, beauty, fitness and overall success departments, also has to deal with stalking, legal disputes, a total lack of privacy and an unnatural level of scrutiny over every single action or word spoken. What constitutes a 'big' problem to one person might be insignificant to another. The most interesting bit is how different people choose to deal with their misfortunes. *That* is what makes the person.

The last ten years have shown me that I am often stronger than I once gave myself credit for. It's probably because I've had to practise quite a lot. When somebody tells me I'm 'brave', I thank them politely, for it's a very kind, well-intentioned sentiment. But I don't ever *feel* brave. Most of the time, I'm actually terrified, but I don't have any other option other than to just crack on with it.

I believe that most people I know, if they were in a similar situation to mine, would respond in the same way, because I see their strength in dealing with non-health challenges. I always hope for the best, whilst preparing for the worst.

Whilst I go through life as a full-time patient, there is ultimately always freedom in how I choose to respond to my situation. Like a liver disease Liam Neeson, I have honed a very particular set of skills which allow me to work through difficulties. I am increasingly confident in my ability to deal with problems, and that sense of self-belief is, I think, one of the most important strengths a person can garner. The narratives which we tell ourselves are powerful; they can help guide us through difficulties and onto happiness again.

Sure, from time to time I can't resist conjuring up an imagined version of what my life would be like if my immune system worked properly. Would I be happier? Would I be living elsewhere, doing more exciting things with my life, stretching my potential more, earning more money? Would I have more friends, a partner, children? If I'm in a negative thought cycle, I'll think the answer is easy: yes, of course, my life would be better.

Yet as I wander through life – more of a tentative crawl, to be honest, stopping for multiple naps en route – the more I realise that everything is a balance. There is good in the bad, and bad in the good. We live in a world where too many things are immediately siloed into one of two camps, without much introspection or interrogation into the middle ground, the nuance. And my life is jam-packed full of nuance.

Chronic illness and me are intrinsically linked. Whilst I don't stride up to people on the street, proffer my hand and introduce myself as Kirsty *'Love Your Liver'* Mills, my autoimmune conditions have made me the person I am today. I'd like to think 19-year-old me would be really proud of her 30-something counterpart.

So, whilst I embark on the remainder of my life sailing in my wee rowing boat across very choppy, shark-infested waters, with no GPS and an out-of-date flare, I've decided to just tighten up my safety-vest as much as possible and sit back to enjoy the fresh air. In the words of one of our generation's finest lyricists, Ronan Keating, life is a rollercoaster. I've just got to ride it.

# ACKNOWLEDGEMENTS

Thank you for taking the time out of your life to read this book. I hope I've managed to convey how chronic illness has, in a roundabout way, been a hugely positive influence on my life. Of course, that life wouldn't be half as great as it is without the support of many people. Thank you to:

Kirsty Ross (as you will always be to me) – for diligently reading my material. You are a wonderful human and a true friend.

Heather – for being an all-round fantastic friend who: inspires me with your volunteering, listens to my rants, is always keen for an exercise class, and is someone I know I can rely on if I need help. They should bottle your attitude and prescribe it on the NHS.

Karen – for being so empathetic and thoughtful, and for always knowing the right thing to say. You constantly inspire me to be a better person.

Ruth – for our evening walks, boxercise classes and weekend lunches which were a steady source of support when I was in Gala. I always hang up after our calls feeling much happier.

Lindsay – for being an amazing sounding board on all life things, but especially on medical shenanigans. You help me more than I think you realise. Also, thanks for single-handedly supporting the French postal system with postcards.

Nicole – for always being there, even from afar, to provide a sensible, thoughtful and intelligent take on virtually any problem.

Fiona – for inspiring me with your light-hearted approach to life…and your endlessly infectious laugh.

Karina – for being a friend who totally gets chronic illness. I think our paths were destined to cross.

(Special mention to all the other lovely ladies – Kirsty, Callie, and Sarah to name but a few - who supported me through my time in the Borders.)

Rhona, Dagne, and Rachael – for your kindness, wisdom, ability to listen and for our lunches and flower workshops.

Becca – for being a likeminded pal since our very first week at Darroch Court. Thank you for your brilliant sense of humour, your ability to keep it real, and for granting me the privilege of reading at your wedding. (And thanks for driving us round Mull.)

Charlotte and Becky – for being caring and thoughtful friends who Zoomed religiously for catchups during Covid.

Gillian – for your ability to make me laugh at mostly everything and anything. It's always a pleasure to catch up in Glasgow. Thank you especially for the Percy Pig memorabilia.

Emma (and all the other ladies who attended my Inverness alopecia support group over the years) – for being a fantastic support network and showing me how incredibly strong people can be.

Special colleagues who have supported me over the years (Sylvia, Paul, Nanette, Jo, KKI Kate, Sean, Brian, Emily D, Michael, Viviane, Clare, GSK Kate, Andy, David, Nicki, Cara,

Steven, Andy, Laura W, Laura M, Lorna, and Sarah) – for encouraging me, reminding me that there is more to life than work, and for making time spent at work more enjoyable.

Shona and Lisa – for being my liver disease inspirations. Words can't describe how much admiration I have for you both and your approach to life.

All the amazing people on the Under 40s Liver WhatsApp chat – for your support during Covid, helping me to feel a little less alone.

Amy and all the other British Liver Trust team members – for being friendly faces and genuinely trying to make life easier for those of us with liver problems.

Dr Alistair MacGilchrist – for helping the 20-year-old who walked cluelessly into hepatology one spring morning and had her entire life flipped upside down. You were calm and kind, and your sage advice (that time tends to heal most things, and that it wouldn't be a good idea to give up my studies) was spot on.

Dr Andrea Broad – for always replying to my queries ASAP and for your honest, *here's-the-situation* approach. It really helps to feel like your doctor is fighting your corner, and you skillfully balance treating me as a patient whilst being fully cognisant of the type of person I am. I appreciate you taking the time to explain the science of what's happening to me (albeit at a high level!), and I consider myself very privileged to have a hepatologist who just *gets* stuff like IUDs and all the other more general life considerations. I think you're a brilliant doctor and I am lucky to have you and the liver nurses on my team.

Dr Tim Gordon-Walker – for being a calming and level-headed presence, as demonstrated at the start of the pandemic when you cheerily advised I simply load up on Netflix recommendations for the foreseeable. I don't envy the decisions you have to make in terms of balancing risks, but I trust your ability to do so, and I think you've done a great job at steering my treatment over the last six years. I'm also always impressed that you remember wee random non-liver facts about me in amongst all your other patients. It's the little things that count, and it's appreciated.

The liver nurses (especially Leighann), the ITR nurses (especially Clare and Sarah-Jane), the medical secretaries (especially Nancy and Mei Lin), the GPs at Nairn Healthcare, Dr Sharkey and Dr Howe, the entire endoscopy unit at Raigmore who are just the best, and the driver who takes bloods to the hospital – for all your help and care over the years. Without your support, I wouldn't be able to live my life.

The anonymous person who kindly donated their blood at the Borders General Hospital – for saving my life.

All the people who went on clinical trials for my medications, and all the people who have had liver disease and lupus before me – for contributing towards scientific knowledge that has helped me to live a better life.

Mrs. Winfield, Miss Philip, Mr. Dawson and Mr. Maclennan – for inspiring and encouraging me as a student.

The many men I've gone on dates with over the years – for teaching me so much more about myself than I could have learned alone. Whilst the dates have not always been what I'd call *fun*, I'm grateful for the experience.

Graham – for all your hard work in creating an awesome cover design.

John – for being the first person to read this all the way through without falling asleep, and for making me laugh.

*Finally, but above all, I would like to thank my family for their love, support, and much-needed reality checks over the course of my life.*

To Poppy – You're the best labrador in the world.

To Emily – You are the kindest, most thoughtful, most fiercely stubborn, funniest, most opposite-to-me-yet-also-the-same-person sister I could ever ask for. I'm so lucky to have a best friend who also shares some DNA, and besides your spectacular ability to mishear song lyrics, my favourite aspect of you is your incredible ability to listen without judgement. You are the only person who can sympathise with what I'm going through whilst knowing when to hold me to account. That balance is so dearly appreciated. It must be difficult to have a sister who often hogs the limelight with the medical stuff, but you've never complained. You're wise beyond your years, and I think you're amazing.

To Mum and Dad – It's not like me, but I don't really have words to express how grateful I am to have been born into your family. Thank you for your wisdom, patience, and guidance in all aspects of my life. I'm sorry to have caused you so much worry, and in many ways it's a cruelty all of its own in having to see your child unwell, but you have never shown me anything other than unwavering support. Without your love, I would not have been able to become the person I'm proud to be today. This book is for you both.

# RESOURCES

For information about liver health, please visit www.britishlivertrust.co.uk. The Trust have a simple health questionnaire to estimate your risk of liver disease.

For information about organ donation, please visit www.organdonation.nhs.uk. Organ donation has the potential to radically change lives. Please have a chat with your loved ones and make them certain about your choices regarding donation.

For information about lupus, please visit www.lupus.org.

For information about alopecia, please visit www.alopecia.org.uk.

Any feedback or corrections are more than welcome; please get in touch via the form on my website (www.kirstymills.org) or by emailing kirstymillswriter@gmail.com.

# REFERENCES


**ON THE ROAD TO DIAGNOSIS**

[i] www.wrenproject.org/who-we-are

[ii] www.lupus.org/resources/what-does-lupus-erythematosus-mean

**ON HOW THE LIVER WORKS…**

[iii] www.britishlivertrust.org.uk/about-us/media-centre/5-facts-about-the-liver/

[iv] Vikramjit Mitra, Jane Metcalf, Functional anatomy and blood supply of the liver, Anaesthesia & Intensive Care Medicine, Volume 13, Issue 2, 2012, Pages 52-53, www.sciencedirect.com/science/article/pii/S1472029911002682

[v] Romer, Alfred Sherwood; Parsons, Thomas S. (1977). *The Vertebrate Body.* Philadelphia, PA: Holt-Saunders International. pp. 354–355.

[vi] www.nottingham.ac.uk/helmopen/rlos/biological-sciences/gastrointestinal-system/liver-anatomy/page_two.html

[vii] Kalra A, Yetiskul E, Wehrle CJ, et al. Physiology, Liver. [Updated 2023 May 1]. Available from: www.ncbi.nlm.nih.gov/books/NBK535438/

[viii] www.my.clevelandclinic.org/health/body/hepatic-veins

[ix] www.hopkinsmedicine.org/health/conditions-and-diseases/liver-anatomy-and-functions

[x] www.e-safe-anaesthesia.org/e_library/02/Liver_physiology_Update_2008.pdf

[xi] Vernon H, Wehrle CJ, Alia VSK, et al. Anatomy, Abdomen and Pelvis: Liver. [Updated 2022 Nov 26]. In: StatPearls [Internet]. Treasure Island (FL): StatPearls Publishing; 2025 Jan-. Available from: www.ncbi.nlm.nih.gov/books/NBK500014

[xii] www.nottingham.ac.uk/helmopen/rlos/biological-sciences/gastrointestinal-system/liver-anatomy

[xiii] www.gastrojournal.org/article/S0016-5085(03)02062-6/fulltext

[xiv] www.michiganmedicine.org/health-lab/what-does-liver-do-and-how-do-i-keep-mine-healthy

[xv] www.columbiasurgery.org/liver/liver-and-its-functions

[xvi] www.nottingham.ac.uk/helmopen/rlos/biological-sciences/gastrointestinal-system/liver-anatomy

[xvii] www.asterlabs.in/resources/blogs/7-most-important-facts-about-liver

[xviii] www.sciencedirect.com/science/article/pii/S155041311730503X

**…AND WHAT HAPPENS WHEN IT DOESN'T**

[xix] www.nhsinform.scot/illnesses-and-conditions/stomach-liver-and-gastrointestinal-tract/liver-disease

[xx] www.britishlivertrust.org.uk/information-and-support/liver-health-2/stages-of-liver-disease/fibrosis

[xxi] www.science.org/doi/10.1126/science.abg4864

[xxii] www.nih.gov/news-events/nih-research-matters/cells-maintain-repair-liver-identified

[xxiii] www.nhsinform.scot/illnesses-and-conditions/stomach-liver-and-gastrointestinal-tract/cirrhosis/#about-cirrhosis

[xxiv] www.medlineplus.gov/ency/article/000489.htm

[xxv] www.liverfoundation.org/about-your-liver/how-liver-diseases-progress/cirrhosis-

severe-scarring
xxvi www.medanta.org/patient-education-blog/10-surprising-facts-about-liver-we-bet-you-didnt-know
xxvii www.britishlivertrust.org.uk/information-and-support/liver-conditions/viralhepatitis
xxviii www.hepctrust.org.uk/find-support/infected-blood-and-blood-products/infected-blood-inquiry
xxix www.britishlivertrust.org.uk/information-and-support/liver-conditions/viralhepatitis
xxx www.britishlivertrust.org.uk/information-and-support/liver-conditions/masld-nafld-and-fatty-liver-disease/
xxxi www.britishlivertrust.org.uk/information-and-support/liver-conditions/masld-nafld-and-fatty-liver-disease
xxxii www.britishlivertrust.org.uk/information-and-support/liver-conditions/primary-biliary-cholangitis
xxxiii www.pscsupport.org.uk/psc-and-other-autoimmune-diseases/pbc-and-psc
xxxiv www.childliverdisease.org/liver-information/childhood-liver-conditions/biliary-atresia
xxxv www.mayoclinic.org/diseases-conditions/wilsons-disease/symptoms-causes
xxxvi www.cysticfibrosis.org.uk/what-is-cystic-fibrosis/how-does-cystic-fibrosis-affect-the-body/symptoms-of-cystic-fibrosis/liver-disease
xxxvii www.britishlivertrust.org.uk/information-and-support/liver-conditions/haemochromatosis
xxxviii www.britishlivertrust.org.uk/information-and-support/liver-conditions/budd-chiari
xxxix www.britishlivertrust.org.uk/information-and-support/liver-conditions/alcohol-related-liver-disease
xl www.nhsbtdbe.blob.core.windows.net/umbraco-assets-corp/36246/nhsbt-united-kingdom-summary-report-mar-25.pdf
xli www.nhsbtdbe.blob.core.windows.net/umbraco-assets-corp/36246/nhsbt-united-kingdom-summary-report-mar-25.pdf
xlii www.britishlivertrust.org.uk/information-and-support/statistics
xliii www.britishlivertrust.org.uk/three-steps-to-love-your-liver
xliv https://britishlivertrust.org.uk/information-and-support/support-for-you/your-stories/anninders-story-i-have-a-liver-condition-called-autoimmune-hepatitis-and-i-know-the-warning-signs-now-and-what-i-have-to-do

**ON MY LIVER HEROES**

xlv www.news-medical.net/health/Hepatology-History.aspx
xlvi www.theguardian.com/science/2020/aug/10/roger-williams-obituary
xlvii www.laskerfoundation.org/an-artist-in-the-operating-room-and-beyond/
xlviii With information from 'Prof' by Om P Sharma
xlix www.britishlivertrust.org.uk/professor-dame-sheila-sherlock-a-life-devoted-to-the-liver/
l www.history.rcplondon.ac.uk/inspiring-physicians/sir-john-mcmichael
li www.ncbi.nlm.nih.gov/pmc/articles/PMC1122088/
lii www.easl.eu/professor-juan-rodes/
liii www.gastrojournal.org/aricle/S0016-5085(17)30336-0/pdf

[liv] www.nobelprize.org/prizes/medicine/1988/elion/biographical/
[lv] www.acs.org/education/whatischemistry/women-scientists/gertrude-elion.html
[lvi] www.pmc.ncbi.nlm.nih.gov/articles/PMC5549009/
[lvii] www.web.archive.org/web/20170308221903/http://old.post-gazette.com/healthscience/20000611starzl2.asp
[lviii] www.doi.org/10.1177/29768675231208426
[lix] www.ncbi.nlm.nih.gov/pmc/articles/PMC8968477
[lx] www.theguardian.com/us-news/2017/mar/05/thomas-starzl-liver-transplant-drug-researcher-dies
[lxi] www.journal-of-hepatology.eu/article/S0168-8278(17)32011-1/
[lxii] www.bbc.co.uk/news/uk-scotland-50572269
[lxiii] www.express.co.uk/life-style/health/182266/Elena-Baltacha-on-her-incurable-liver-disease

**ON MEDICS**
[lxiv] Fitch, Tad; Layton, J. Kent; Wormstedt, Bill (2012). On A Sea of Glass: The Life & Loss of the R.M.S. Titanic. Amberley Books.

**ON DATING, SINGLEDOM AND SELF-RESPECT**
[lxv] www.bannerjones.co.uk/resources/chronic-illness-and-divorce
[lxvi] www.pharm.or.jp/eng/em-medicine.html
[lxvii] www.sciencedirect.com/topics/neuroscience/tacrolimus
[lxviii] www.pubchem.ncbi.nlm.nih.gov/compound/Tacrolimus
[lxix] www.britishlivertrust.org.uk/information-and-support/statistics
[lxx] www.britishlivertrust.org.uk/liver-disease-is-now-the-biggest-cause-of-death-in-those-aged-between-35-49-years-old-new-report-reveals/

**ON BABIES (OR LACK THEREOF)**
[lxxi] www.hematology.org/education/patients/anemia/pregnancy
[lxxii] www.nhs.uk/conditions/gestational-diabetes/
[lxxiii] www.npeu.ox.ac.uk/ukoss/completed-surveillance/cirrhosis-in-pregnancy

**ON MENTAL HEALTH**
[lxxiv] www.doi.org/10.3389/fpsyt.2020.00451
[lxxv] Viktor E Frankl, 'Man's Search For Meaning'

www.ingramcontent.com/pod-product-compliance
Ingram Content Group UK Ltd.
Pitfield, Milton Keynes, MK11 3LW, UK
UKHW041905040226
10508UKWH00002B/293

9 781036 929374